The Bitter Sweet

The Bitter Sweet

RECOGNIZING AND RESOLVING
THE SUGAR CRISIS

• • •

Harry G. Preuss, MD

ISBN: 1544239270
ISBN 13: 9781544239279
Library of Congress Control Number: 2017903573
CreateSpace Independent Publishing Platform
North Charleston, South Carolina

Dedication

This book is dedicated to my wife Bonnie (Veronica Coleman Preuss) who as many of my colleagues have wisely perceived is my "strength" and to my four wonderful, supporting children who have brought me much pride: Mary Beth Preuss Carney, Jeffrey Michael Preuss M.D., Christopher David Preuss and Michael David Preuss.

Disclaimer

• • •

THE INFORMATION IN THIS BOOK is intended to be educational, not to diagnose or treat any known or suspected disease. The author recommends consulting a qualified medical professional for assessment, diagnosis, and treatment of any suspected or known medical condition, or symptoms that may be an indicator of declining health. Any recommendations for diet, exercise, or the use of dietary supplements is presented only for informational purposes and is not intended to substitute for competent medical advice.

Books Written for Public by Dr. Preuss

Preuss HG, Adderly B: The Prostate Cure. Crown Publishers, Inc. NewYork, NY, 1998.

PREUSS HG, KONNO S: MAITAKE Magic, Freedom Press, Topanga CA, 2002.

Preuss HG, Gottlieb W: The Natural Fat Loss Pharmacy Broadway Books, New York, NY, pp 1-260, 2007.

Table of Contents

Disclaimer ·vii
Introduction · xiii

Chapter 1   The Dangers of Modern Life ·1
Chapter 2   Why Too Much Sugar Is Harmful · · · · · · · · · · · · · · · · ·7
Chapter 3   Lifestyle Solutions ·16
Chapter 4   What Is a Healthy Weight? ·22
Chapter 5   Poor Choices of Foods and Drinks · · · · · · · · · · · · · · ·30
Chapter 6   What to Eat and Drink for Better Health · · · · · · · · · · · · ·37
Chapter 7   Easy Ways to be More Active ·43
Chapter 8   Dietary Supplements: Aids in Prevention · · · · · · · · · · · · ·48
Chapter 9   Improving Insulin Sensitivity with Chromium · · · · · · · · · ·53
Chapter 10   Supplements that Block Sugar and Starch Absorption · · · ·63
Chapter 11   Fat Burners and Other Aids ·71
Chapter 12   The Practical Plan ·76

References ·85
Author Biography · 101
Selected Author Bibliography · 105

Introduction

• • •

I BELIEVE MOST OF CIVILIZATION is in the midst of a "sugar crisis" that is universally affecting long-term, general health in an unfortunate manner. The crisis-producing sugar is sucrose, a combination of two simpler bound sugars I'm sure you've heard of -- glucose and fructose. If you're befuddled by the terminology, sucrose in everyday life is simply common "table sugar."

To emphasize my convictions, I frequently refer to sucrose as a "bitter sweet." On the sweet side, it provides instant, satisfying pleasure to our senses. On the bitter side, in addition to supplying too many calories without nutritional benefits, it can encourage weight gain, prevent weight loss, and contribute in a major fashion to diabetes, heart disease, and premature aging.

In support of my catch phrase, the following fact is undeniably bittersweet: The rise of obesity and diabetes coincides closely with increased consumption of sugar. Always a desired food, sugar was once too expensive for most individuals but now, it is readily available in thousands of foods and beverages. Sodas, candy, sweet snacks, and desserts are obvious ones, but sugar is also in many other processed foods, such as soups, sauces, ketchup, cereals, frozen meals, nutrition bars, and many canned foods. These items are convenient, usually inexpensive, plentiful, and when eaten in excess — and I'm not saying this just to be dramatic — deadly.

Often, I am asked, "How did you get started in medical research, and why?" Being a fan of Socrates, the Greek philosopher, I've always tried to adhere to his adage to "know thyself," and I had doubts about my ability to be original in thought. It was one thing to obtain much knowledge from others and use it properly in my college and medical training, but could I develop original concepts?

Accordingly, after three years of clinical preparation at Vanderbilt University Medical Center in Nashville, Tennessee, I decided that I would be a better physician with some research training. I also wanted to test my abilities to develop original ideas in medicine. So, I returned to my medical school, Cornell Medical Center in New York City, to work under the tutelage of Dr. Robert F. Pitts. At that time, he was a world leader in studying the kidney and nervous system — an international medical "celebrity," so to speak — and someone I highly admired during my student days.

Upon my arrival, I became aware of a problem Dr. Pitts had encountered in his study of kidney function. He had observed a phenomenon that defied current understanding of exactly how this organ works. Over the next few months, this particular problem was discussed again and again at departmental gatherings. As a neophyte should, I spent much time in the library, and while reading a scientific paper, lights went off in my head. I told Dr. Pitts that I may have found the answer to his dilemma and lo and behold, I was right. I had identified a mechanism that shed light on what had mystified my mentor.

During the next year, I performed much research on my own, still uncertain of my ability to discover or formulate original scientific ideas — but my confidence would get a boost. By the time I was leaving Cornell, Dr. Pitts told me that my research, which gave us a better understanding of how the kidney works, had given him new ideas to pursue for the rest of his working years. This acknowledgement was a special moment, and I left my postdoctoral training feeling reassured that I could perform important, innovative research.

I then went to Georgetown Medical Center for more training in clinical medicine, and continued the kidney research I had begun at Cornell. However, when I initially submitted my findings to medical journals, reviewers derided my conclusions. And then, I experienced some unexpected satisfaction. At a scientific conference in Montreal, Dr. Hans Krebs, recipient of a Nobel Prize for discoveries we refer to as the "Krebs cycle," said from the stage that my basic theories about kidney function were correct. From that moment on, I had even more confidence in my original thinking, and began writing more papers and giving presentations in nephrology, the medical specialty that deals with the kidneys. These initial experiences gave me more confidence to break new ground in other areas of health.

My study of nutrition was sparked in the late 1970s, when my daughter asked for help with a science project. Using rats, we found that sugar-sweetened drinks could significantly raise systolic blood pressure – the top number — and in 1980, the findings were published in a scientific journal. From then on, I spent a good deal of time examining the detrimental effects of sugar and ways to overcome sugar-related maladies.

In the years since then, clinical studies in my lab have demonstrated that eating too many refined carbohydrates, especially sugar (and high fructose corn syrup), leads to insulin resistance. This phenomenon, which I'll explain in more detail in the first few chapters of the book, is a major trigger for many harmful changes, including rising blood pressure, rising blood glucose, high triglycerides, low HDL cholesterol, weight gain, and inflammation. A combination of these factors is known as metabolic syndrome. It affects three critical health areas: premature aging, obesity, and development of type 2 diabetes. Consequences include increased risk for heart disease, joint problems, and development and worsening of certain cancers. How much sugar do you have to eat or drink to face these health risks? Sadly, amounts that are commonly consumed in the Western diet are sufficient.

For a long time, it wasn't easy for me to get across the problems that dietary sugar could initiate, because there was such a strong belief in the medical community that sugar was relatively benign, and that saturated fats were the root of all evil. There were some courageous individuals who did not adhere to the conventional view, but they tended to be highly criticized. One was the late Dr. Mary Enig. I remember many enlightening conversations with her. A good friend, Mary had observed for many years that saturated fats were not as dangerous as proposed, but that "trans fats" in our cooking oils and margarines (partially hydrogenated oils) posed the real health problems. After one of our discussions, I remember going home and telling my wife we were switching back to butter.

I always admired Mary's show of courage in facing up to criticism, and her determination to present the facts helped me deal with backlash that I, too, experienced. One such instance occurred at a meeting of the National Cholesterol Education Program (NCEP), a program to reduce heart disease, under the National Institutes of Health. The meeting took place some years ago, when I was a member of the NCEP advisory council, and the adverse effects of sugar were not recognized in conventional medical circles. During a breakout session, I commented that some statements made by NCEP were increasing obesity in the nation, because they were directing people to avoid saturated fats and instead, consume more sugar and refined carbohydrates. Afterward, addressing the general meeting, the session coordinator presented my statement almost as a joke. However, by the end of the meeting, it was decided to have a group look further into the issue. It was an uncomfortable situation but I felt I had made a dent in the sugar-versus-fat debate. Today, excess sugar is recognized as a serious problem, but its overconsumption still drives disease.

Treatment for sugar-induced maladies has produced some useful and perhaps surprising information. For obesity and diabetes, the history of prescription drugs is often one of disaster, due to adverse reactions. Fortunately, we have also learned that there are many safer dietary supplements to help solve the problem, in conjunction with lifestyle changes. Claims about supplements are sometimes over-hyped, but there is good evidence that certain ones have the ability to overcome insulin resistance or reduce the harm from excess carbohydrates. Two natural, safe supplement categories I favor are "insulin sensitizers," such as chromium, and "carbohydrate blockers," such as bean and hibiscus extracts, and l-arabinose.

Today, there are more health books than at any other time in our history, but there is still much confusion about what is a "healthy" diet. My purpose in writing this book is not only to make readers aware of the health problems that too much sugar and other, well-liked, refined carbohydrates can cause or advance, but also to provide evidence-based information about simple, safe ways to reduce the damage and perhaps prevent chronic disorders like obesity, diabetes, and cardiovascular diseases. I hope this book is helpful in your quest for a longer, healthier lifespan.

CHAPTER 1
The Dangers of Modern Life

• • •

EVER SINCE THE DISCOVERY OF sugar, we've been enamored with it. At first, it was only available to the privileged few but as supply increased, people devoured more and more — often far too much. This widespread popularity no doubt emanates from its pleasurable, sweet taste but other consequences are anything but sweet.

Today, we have global epidemics of obesity and diabetes that I believe are due, at least to some extent, to excess consumption of sugar. In turn, obesity and diabetes are closely linked to heart disease and other disabling and deadly medical conditions. As the final straw, addiction, a word that makes most people shudder, may also play a significant role in the attraction to sugar. Such negative information has led to my belief that it is, indeed, a bitter sweet.

The knowledge that sugar can harm human health has been available for a long time. I became aware of this in the late 1970s, while researching the effects of sugar on blood pressure and reviewing the work of Dr. John Yudkin, a brilliant British physician who was trying to warn the world about the danger of sugar. Dr. Yudkin's extensive research provided solid evidence that consuming too much sugar leads to medical maladies but unfortunately, he was so vehemently criticized as to be virtually forgotten. Since then, there have been many corroborating studies, including a few dozen of my own.

I believe the time has come to recognize the danger of excess sugar: increasing rates of diabetes, obesity, hypertension, a variety of cardiovascular disorders, and other related health woes. The statistics are shocking. The World Health Organization estimates that today, there are about four times as many people with diabetes as there were a few decades ago, despite many medical advances. To be more precise with numbers, in 1980, there were 108 million adults worldwide with diabetes and now, there are at least 422 million.

The Food and Agriculture Organization of the United Nations reports that globally, more than one in three people are overweight and more than one in ten are obese, and the figures are much higher in some areas. Among major countries, Mexico has the highest rate of obesity, with 32.8 percent of adults being obese, and the United States is a close second, with 31.8 percent. The close association of obesity and diabetes has led to the term "diabesity" to emphasize the link between the two concurrent epidemics.

In the past, there were disagreements among scientists about how much harm sugar really causes. However, in more recent times, there has been less doubt in the minds of many that too much can lead to harmful health problems. Such problems coincide with the obvious fact that more and more processed foods and drinks with added sugar have become conveniently available in every corner of our lives, in many schools, work places, restaurants, stores, movie theaters, and anywhere else we go for entertainment.

AN OLD PROBLEM

Starting in the 17th century, sugar began to be widely cultivated on plantations in the Caribbean and became available to many Europeans. In 1675, a British doctor noted that the urine of people with diabetes had a sweet smell but sugars like sucrose (what we call "table sugar"), and its simpler components, fructose and glucose, were not clearly identified as being harmful or related to diabetes until the 20th century.

A Harvard doctor who was a pioneer in treating diabetes, Elliot Joslin, observed an 80-percent increase in deaths from diabetes between 1900 and 1915. Joslin, who founded the famous Joslin Diabetes Center, called diabetes "a penalty of obesity." In the early 1900s, obesity was viewed as a product of modern life, with food being more plentiful, automation replacing much physical labor, and more sucrose in people's diets. (Unfortunately, we still haven't solved these problems.) Despite the fact that a few forward-thinking doctors were connecting sugar intake, obesity, and diabetes nearly 100 years ago, these ideas were not truly accepted by the majority over the following decades.

DEBATE ABOUT SUGAR AND FAT

During World War I, there were marked improvements in health among the British population: significantly less obesity, diabetes, and heart disease. These temporary benefits coincided with scarcities of both sugar and fat, and when scientists later began examining the matter, a war of ideas ensued. Some argued that the main reason for the healthy turnabout was less sugar consumption, while others concluded it was less fat intake. While many took one side or the other, a combination of less sugar and fat consumption was also favored. A similar pattern occurred after World War II and the scientific debate about the relative importance of sugar and fat continued.

From the 1950s onward, as all types of food became plentiful, research findings by an increasing number of scientists favored a premise that sugar was largely responsible for increasing rates of diabetes and heart disease. Studies also demonstrated that sugar leads to high blood pressure, which raises risk for both heart disease and strokes. One review, in 1974, noted that the amount of sugar in the average Western diet was seven times what it used to be, and that this was a major reason for rising blood pressure in the Western world.

Despite solid evidence that excess dietary sugar is harmful to general health, more doctors, scientists, and nutritionists focused virtually exclusively on the proposal that eating too much fat, especially saturated fat, was by far the major dietary nemesis in public health. So, fat won the "importance debate," hands down. Saturated fat became universally recognized as the unhealthiest ingredient in food, one to be avoided as much as possible.

In the United States, the government began recommending a low-fat diet, with many of the low-fat foods containing refined carbohydrates and lots of sugar. In 1991, A US government report encouraged manufacturers to double the number of such food products and recommended a high-carbohydrate diet. Unfortunately, a number of refined carbohydrates are just as harmful as sugar, and such foods often combine large quantities of these two ingredients.

The same theory became adopted in other countries and as a result, low-fat foods have been widely promoted as being healthy. Yet, because they provide an excess of sugar and refined carbohydrates, we now suspect strongly that they are the main dietary reason why obesity and diabetes have continued to rise as never before. Ironically, rather than improving health, low-fat processed foods may have helped triple obesity, dramatically increased diabetes, and promoted heart disease.

HIDDEN INDUSTRY INFLUENCE

While the epidemic of obesity and diabetes has been raging, there have been physicians and researchers, and I include myself in this group, who have continued to present evidence of sugar being the most harmful, widely used ingredient in our food. Change has been slow, but it has been taking place. In 2015, the US government issued dietary guidelines that no longer set limits on fat in the diet but did recommend limiting added sugar.

Why did it take so long for the dangers of sugar to begin to be recognized widely? There are charges that the sugar industry played a prominent role in influencing the scientific data to prevent a decrease in the use of sugar. For example, in 2016, a group of independent researchers documented one significant example of how industry helped establish the false notion that fat causes heart disease but sugar is not harmful. Their research was published in a respected medical journal, *JAMA Internal Medicine*.

This is what the independent researchers documented: In 1965, the publication of three scientific articles, showing that sugar caused heart disease, made headlines in an influential New York daily newspaper. Two days later, the Sugar Research Foundation (now called the World Sugar Research Organization) approved funding for a project to discredit these data. The foundation paid leading scientists at the Harvard University School of Public Health Nutrition Department to produce articles showing that sugar was not harmful after all, and that fat was the real cause of heart disease. These scientists compiled earlier studies in a manner that led to a false conclusion, and their work was published in a top journal, the *New England Journal of Medicine*.

At that time, the journal did not require disclosure of how studies were funded, so the connection of the study authors to the sugar industry was hidden. Since then, this and other journals routinely require that funding for a study or any other potential conflicts of interest must be disclosed by authors of scientific articles.

The 2016 study is only one example of how scientific data and dietary recommendations have been influenced by industry, and it isn't the only reason why the danger of too much sugar intake was ignored for decades. However, it certainly helps to explain why science was ignored and low-fat foods, high in harmful sugar and refined carbohydrates, were promoted as the healthy way to eat. Nevertheless, human beings like sugar and generally don't need to be persuaded to eat it. In the last 50 years, mass production and marketing of convenient, inexpensive, high-sugar foods have prevailed.

CHAPTER 2

Why Too Much Sugar Is Harmful

• • •

BEFORE DIABETES AND HEART DISEASE develop, gradual alterations take place in the human body over a period of time. Some of these, such as blood pressure changes, are well recognized, routinely measured, and can be treated. More recently, many believe that elevated fasting glucose concentrations, even within ranges designated as normal, may also be a basic and important sign foretelling harmful changes that could occur over time. It's important to note that the circulating concentration of glucose, the commonly measured sugar in blood, is influenced to a great extent by diet.

To clarify some important terminology, most scientists and nutritionists would concur that when speaking of food, "sugar" refers to sucrose, which is a combination of glucose and fructose bound together. Sucrose is also typically called "table sugar." When discussing food or beverages, I'll use the terms "sugar" and "sucrose" interchangeably. However, when there is a discussion of "blood sugar," meaning sugar circulating in the blood, this typically refers to glucose, because glucose is the primary form of sugar that is found and measured in our bodies. In the rest of the book, I'll use the term "glucose" when referring to its levels in the blood.

After we eat sucrose or most starches, enzymes in the gastrointestinal tract break down larger units into smaller ones, referred to as "simple sugars." In the case of sucrose, the enzymes break apart the bond that holds glucose and fructose together. These smaller units can then be absorbed, and glucose levels rise measurably in the blood that circulates through the body.

As a technical note, another, very popular sweetener, high fructose corn syrup, does not have to work in the same way. Like sucrose, high fructose corn syrup is made up of glucose and fructose, but these are not chemically bound together. Rather, they are free, unattached simple sugars and do not need to be broken down by enzymes before being absorbed.

Glucose in blood is an essential type of fuel. As blood circulates, the glucose is transported through the blood to cells, where it is primarily used to generate energy. However, the process begins to cause unwanted health disturbances when blood levels of glucose are repeatedly too high. Today, it is commonly agreed that fasting blood glucose levels in a range of 100-125 mg/dl, often described as a "prediabetic" state, provide a warning sign to do something to remedy this situation. Persistent fasting glucose levels above 125 mg/dl are diagnosed as diabetes and demand urgent treatment. Some statistics show just how dangerous this situation can become.

According to the World Health Organization, diabetes caused 1.5 million deaths in 2012, but deaths from higher-than-optimal blood glucose caused another 2.2 million deaths, by increasing risk for heart disease and other conditions. Close to half of these deaths occurred before age 70, and I believe many could have been prevented, or lives could have been improved with a healthier diet and lifestyle.

WHERE THE PROBLEM BEGINS

When everything is functioning as it should, this is roughly what happens after consuming sugars and/or certain carbohydrates: Levels of circulating glucose rise. In response, insulin is released. Insulin is a hormone, which acts like a messenger by telling cells to absorb glucose from the blood so that they can use it to generate energy. The glucose is the essential fuel for muscles, the brain, and a variety of other cells in the body. Once cells have absorbed the glucose, the concentration in the bloodstream decreases.

This pattern of higher blood glucose, insulin secretion, absorption of glucose by cells, and lower glucose levels takes place each time we eat sugar, starches, or a combination of the two. It's designed to maintain a healthy balance of fuel for energy. As wonderful as this system is, there are limits to its capabilities. In other words, the system can be abused and unfortunately, the abuse arises within us. Eating too much sugar and starch disrupts the normal process and starts a series of damaging re-actions. Among these is "insulin resistance," where the usual effects of insulin are impaired and it takes more to accomplish the same effect on glucose transport.

As an analogy, imagine this. In a healthy person, insulin is a messenger delivering packages of glucose to the doors of cells, particularly in the muscles, fat, and liver. Insulin knocks on the doors, the cell doors open, the packages are accepted, and the messenger goes away. When things start to go wrong, insulin knocks on the doors but only some answer and fully open the door. This situation, where many cells refuse to open the door or do so incompletely, is called – maybe you guessed it — "insulin resistance." It is a common, unfortunate response to eating too much sugar and other carbohydrates, especially refined carbohydrates. It's important to note that insulin resistance is the first step in the direction of full-blown type 2 diabetes, the most common form of diabetes. Another generally accepted fact is that insulin resistance is more likely to develop as an individual gets older.

The human body is amazing. When certain organs or tissues don't respond to a hormone normally, it can produce more of that hormone in an attempt to compensate. In other words, the appearance of more messengers makes up, at least initially, for a decreased response. The hormonal systems affecting the thyroid and adrenals are examples of such compensatory responses, and the glucose-insulin system is another.

As a person keeps eating too much sugar and refined carbohydrates, such as white flour, the ability of the cells to respond properly is diminished. To compensate, more and more insulin messengers deliver glucose packages to the doors of cells. While this may help temporarily, as time passes, this compensatory ability decreases. Soon, there are many messengers holding glucose packages, unable to deliver them, and levels of glucose in the blood stabilize at higher levels.

Another bad development is this: The circulating levels of insulin mirror those of glucose in that they remain too high as well. Levels of both become "hyper," meaning abnormally high. Unfortunately, both hyperglycemia — high glucose — and hyperinsulinemia — high insulin — are bad for our health.

How Things Get Worse – Onset of Diabetes

If insulin resistance is not reversed by a healthy diet and lifestyle, the next step works like this: For a while, extra messengers enable more doors to be opened, glucose enters cells, and elevated levels of blood glucose go down, but characteristically stabilize at a higher level than at the start, as do circulating insulin levels. This pattern repeats over time as excess sugars or carbohydrates are eaten. However, it's a struggle, requiring extra insulin to be produced each time to overcome resistance from cells. Slowly but surely, both glucose and insulin continue to gradually increase their circulating concentrations – much to the detriment of many organ systems, especially the cardiovascular system. If there are no changes in the diet, the body will eventually become unable to keep producing additional insulin, above levels that are already elevated. At that point, blood glucose will rise to levels classified as diabetes.

METABOLIC SYNDROME

In the eyes of many specialists in the field, including myself, insulin resistance is a major trigger for an array of harmful health maladies known in medicine as "metabolic syndrome." This state increases risks for diabetes, heart disease, and stroke. The word "metabolic" refers to processes that take place in a human body all the time and are part of its normal function. In metabolic syndrome, some of those processes are not working correctly, and this leads to a variety of diseases.

More precisely, metabolic syndrome means a person has three or more of these characteristics:

- A large waistline or belly, or an apple-shaped body. Excess fat in the stomach area is more dangerous than fat in other parts of the body.
- High fasting blood glucose or requires medication to control blood glucose. Fasting blood glucose is measured with a blood test.
- High blood pressure or requires medication to control blood pressure.

- High triglycerides or the individual requires medication to treat high triglycerides. These are a type of fat found in the blood, often measured at the same time as total cholesterol
- Low levels of HDL cholesterol or the individual requires medication to treat low HDL. HDL is often described as "good cholesterol," because it helps to remove cholesterol from arteries.

This may seem complicated but there is a simple lesson to be learned. I believe preventing or reversing insulin resistance can help stop or at least reduce these disturbing developments.

A Breakthrough Study of Blood Glucose

A number of different blood tests can be used to identify insulin resistance. Among these, fasting blood glucose is a simple one. A sample of blood is taken after the person has not eaten or had anything to drink for at least eight hours, and the blood is analyzed for levels of glucose, measured in milligrams per deciliter, abbreviated mg/dl. In medicine, a level of 100 to 125 mg/dl is defined as "prediabetic," meaning diabetes has not developed yet but is more likely to do so in the future. Readings consistently above 125 mg/dl define diabetes. Below 100 mg/dl is considered "normal." These data are relevant for type 2 diabetes, the most common form.

Where glucose levels are prediabetic or diabetic, insulin resistance is present. However, most medical professionals do not realize that insulin resistance, and harm, probably begin in the higher ranges of what is considered "normal," meaning even below 100 mg/dl. Today, many experts believe that we should keep fasting glucose levels as low as possible, below 85 mg/dl, as long as there are no adverse effects. I believe there is good evidence to support this lower target level.

I often give lectures on this topic to doctors, researchers, and government experts who develop policies on nutrition and health, and find that many highly-educated people are not aware of the most current research on this subject. At many of my recent lectures, some health professionals have been surprised by the information I've presented and which I'm about to share with you.

My colleagues and I did a study with data obtained from nearly 300 "healthy people." We examined results from all the major types of medical tests that are used to determine risks for diabetes and heart disease, including all the characteristics of metabolic syndrome I've listed above. All the people in the study had blood glucose levels in a non-diabetic range, as defined in medicine today (125 mg/dl or lower). Nevertheless, even though they were not diabetic, the higher their blood glucose, the more likely they were to have excess body fat, high blood pressure, high triglycerides, low HDL, and other signs of risk for diabetes and heart disease.

Worth emphasizing, based on the research, I postulate that the higher the fasting glucose concentration, even when considering only the non-diabetic range, the greater the intensity of insulin resistance and its effects. These same, significant correlations existed with circulating insulin levels and A1C, the measure of longer-term levels of blood glucose. These findings suggest that controlling insulin resistance is an important key to a healthy life.

THE DEADLY TRIANGLE

The simple illustration below summarizes a most important principal emanating from my research – the "deadly triangle."

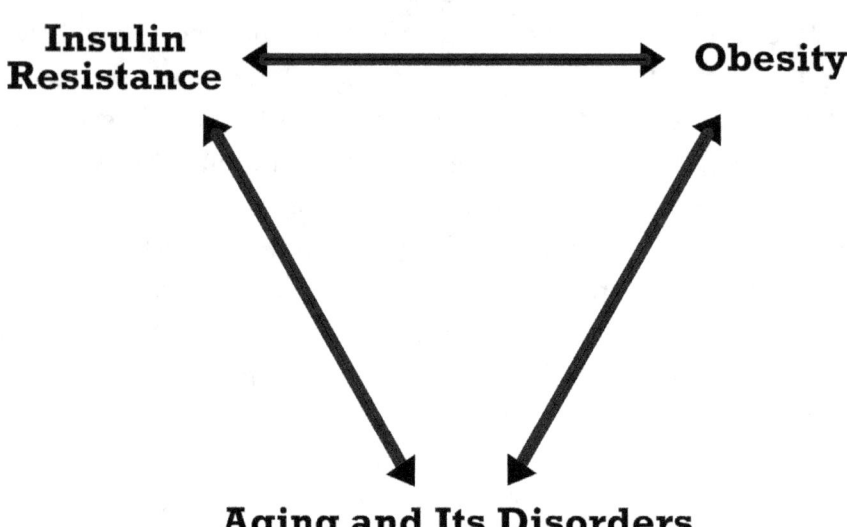

The Deadly Triangle

Insulin Resistance ⟵⟶ **Obesity**

Aging and Its Disorders

Each of the three elements, insulin resistance, obesity, and aging, drive one another. Halting or slowing these elements, even at one point of the triangle, would be beneficial. We can't stop ourselves from getting older, but we can attempt to obtain a healthier and longer lifespan by doing these things:

- favorably changing our diets, by lowering overall intake of calories and refined carbohydrates while maintaining or increasing fiber intake to generally recommended levels
- improving our exercise programs, as exercise can lower body fat and insulin resistance

   ❋   taking supplements that aid in improving body composition and preventing or overcoming insulin resistance

I believe these three steps can help to slow, reduce, and maybe even prevent many chronic disabilities associated with aging. While such a task over the long haul would require some effort, recognizing this simple concept may give impetus to those willing to make important lifestyle changes over a lifetime.

CHAPTER 3
Lifestyle Solutions

• • •

WE OFTEN HEAR ABOUT THE need for a "healthy lifestyle," but what does that mean? Lifestyle is a combination of things we do, or don't do on most days. Some of these affect our health for better or worse. Eating foods that contain a lot of vitamins and minerals can contribute to good health. Drinking a lot of soda or alcoholic drinks, and smoking are associated with bad effects on health. Not being physically active and not getting enough sleep may also detract from our health.

All together, these things are part of a lifestyle and are capable of making a big difference in whether we're healthy or not. There is no guarantee that we will never get sick but on the positive side, we have a lot of control over some of the most common chronic maladies, such as obesity, diabetes, and heart disease.

Take obesity as an example of a controllable plight. To state the obvious, excess body fat is not healthy for reasons other than appearance. Sometimes, being overweight can be a side effect of medications or an underlying medical condition but most of the time, it is a result of poor dietary and exercise habits. The bottom line is that insulin resistance makes it easier to gain weight in the form of fat, and excess body fat contributes to insulin resistance. One drives the other.

On the other hand, weight loss can enhance insulin sensitivity to some extent, and overcoming insulin resistance assists in maintaining healthier levels of body fat. Thus, normalizing one state improves the other and in practical terms, the right lifestyle changes can help solve these inter-related dilemmas.

How much body weight is too much? Opinions can vary in different cultures, and I'll talk more about this in the next chapter. First, I'd like to illustrate the power of an optimal lifestyle to beneficially influence our health, especially when it comes to diabetes and heart disease.

TYPES OF DIABETES

Three different types of diabetes are generally recognized. The most common form and the one discussed here, type 2 diabetes, is principally a severe form of insulin resistance that can largely be influenced favorably with proper diet and exercise. In some cases, the disease may also be virtually reversed, at least to some extent, in the same way. Between 90 and 95 percent of all diabetes in the world is type 2.

Another type, gestational diabetes, may sometimes develop during pregnancy. It is usually temporary if properly treated.

Type 1 diabetes is a condition where there is an inability to produce insulin. It is usually diagnosed in childhood and is believed to have a genetic cause. People with type 1 diabetes must use insulin to control their blood glucose, and there is no known cure. This form of diabetes is often said to be "insulin dependent," unlike type 2 diabetes which, more often than not, is "non-insulin dependent." Although a healthy lifestyle can improve overall well-being, it cannot prevent or reverse type 1 diabetes.

Worldwide, it's estimated that between 5 and 10 percent of people with diabetes have the type 1 form of the disease.

In discussing diabetes prevention in this text, I am referring to the more common type 2 diabetes. Worth emphasizing, studies show that lifestyle changes can often decrease risk for type 2 diabetes, while reducing risk for heart disease at the same time.

DIABETES PREVENTION

Results from the biggest investigation of diabetes prevention, called the Diabetes Prevention Program, or DPP, were published in 2002 in the *New England Journal of Medicine*. The study examined more than 3,200 adults and compared the effects of diet, exercise, and/or a widely used medical drug, metformin, as ways to prevent diabetes.

The study was performed in the United States, with the support of the National Institutes of Health, and included people of many different cultural backgrounds. Nearly half the people in the study were Hispanic, Latino, African American, Alaska Native, American Indian, Asian American, or Pacific Islanders. The common denominator was that all were overweight and prediabetic, meaning they had levels of blood glucose that were elevated, putting them at high risk of developing diabetes, but not high enough to be diabetic at the start of the study.

The DPP study proved two very important points. It established that diabetes could be prevented in some people who were already at high risk for the disease, and that improved lifestyle (diet and exercise) was a more effective therapeutic measure than the medical drug tested.

People in the study were divided into three groups: Those taking a dummy pill, also called a placebo, those taking metformin, a medical drug, and those following a lifestyle program of proper diet and exercise. For the lifestyle group, the aim was to lose seven percent of initial body weight. To give an illustration, if someone weighed 200 pounds, or 91 kilos, the aim was to lose 14 pounds, or about 6.5 kilos. Complementing a prescribed dietary regimen, the lifestyle program included 150 minutes of exercise per week. As an example of how to do this, 150 minutes per week may be accomplished with 30 minutes of exercise on five days of the week.

These were some of the results:

* People following the lifestyle program reduced their risk for diabetes by an average of 58 percent. Among those who were at least 60 years old, risk was reduced even more, by 71 percent.
* The lifestyle program was effective for all those who followed it.
* Losing between 5 and 7 percent of the initial body weight reduced risk for diabetes.
* People taking the medical drug, metformin, decreased their risk for diabetes by an average of only 31 percent, and some people did not benefit at all.
* The medical drug was more helpful for younger people but was not as effective for those age 60 and older.
* The drug did not help prevent diabetes in people who were genetically at the highest risk.
* The lifestyle program continued to be effective in preventing many cases of diabetes for at least 10 years.

There was one other very important outcome. Compared to the drug, the diet and exercise program was more effective in reducing blood pressure and other risk factors for heart disease. This was the largest study showing that diet and exercise can prevent diabetes. Corroborating this study, there are many others with similar positive outcomes. To the best of my knowledge, no one has ever challenged the fact that lifestyle changes are the best-known way to prevent diabetes.

HEART DISEASE

Diabetes doubles the risk for heart disease and strokes, conditions causing nearly one in three of all deaths worldwide. In addition, the World Health Organization estimates that globally, high blood pressure, closely linked to insulin resistance and type 2 diabetes, is responsible for many more deaths, because high blood pressure on its own increases risk for heart disease, strokes, kidney disease, and vision loss.

In medicine today, the causes behind most cases of high blood pressure are "unknown," partially because evidence about the dangers of sugar are overlooked. In the large DPP study above, diet and exercise reduced not only circulating glucose concentrations but also blood pressure. Other studies have found that before diabetes develops, rising levels of blood glucose lead to rising levels of blood pressure. Consequently, lowering blood glucose with diet and exercise to improve insulin sensitivity could potentially help many people with "unknown" causes of blood pressure, by reducing their risks for heart disease and strokes.

There is strong evidence that eating too much sugar contributes to high blood pressure, obesity, harmful levels of cholesterol, and high triglycerides. These are all part of the dangerous metabolic syndrome described in the last chapter.

THE IMPORTANCE OF SLEEP

It may surprise you that sleep is an important part of a healthy lifestyle. Studies show that not getting enough sleep makes it more likely that people will have a bigger appetite, eat too much, become insulin resistant, gain weight, develop diabetes and heart disease, and suffer from premature death.

The first study to show a connection between sleep and early death was published in 1964 and looked at more than one million adults of all ages. Since then, hundreds of studies have looked at how sleep influences the health risks I have been describing. All together, these studies have looked at more than 600,000 children and adults, ranging in ages from 2 to 102. They show that too little sleep, and sometimes too much, leads to obesity, diabetes, and other problems. Between 7 and 9 hours of sleep for adults, and at least 10 for children, are considered optimum amounts of sleep for most.

Consequently, in addition to developing a proper exercise routine and eating in a way that prevents insulin resistance and weight gain, a healthy lifestyle includes getting enough sleep.

CHAPTER 4
What Is a Healthy Weight?

• • •

BODY WEIGHT HAS BEEN VIEWED in different ways during the course of history. Before food began to be produced in mass during the last century, it was a scarce commodity for many people. The wealthy could afford to eat more and often gained weight and so, being overweight became a sign of wealth. In contrast, poor people had little to eat and were often in danger of starvation. In fact, many did die through starvation. Consequently, being thin became a sign of poverty and ill health, but things have changed dramatically with the passage of time.

Today, there is an abundance of convenient, relatively inexpensive processed foods and beverages marketed throughout the world on a massive scale. Unfortunately, these are typically high in calories, often high in sugar, and generally contain low levels of nutrients. As a result, they contribute to obesity, a condition that has become a global problem among adults and children.

Many health departments of various governments, and international organization such as the World Health Organization, have initiated campaigns to try to solve the problem of obesity. Despite this, some cultures do not view being overweight as a bad thing. In fact, some parents mistakenly believe that if their children appear plump, this is a sign of good health. On the other hand, there is a contrasting perspective in other locations. In some Western countries today, a concern persists that showing thin women in popular magazines allows a false impression of what an ideal woman should look like, and that this portrayal may lead to harmful attempts to become too thin.

I recognize that there are cultural differences in what is considered a desirable body weight. I do not intend to judge different cultural ideals. As a doctor and researcher, my concern is only with the effect of surplus body fat on health. There is reasonable scientific evidence that when body weight is too high, it significantly increases risk for diabetes, heart disease, osteoarthritis and other joint problems, and even some cancers, including endometrial, breast, ovarian, prostate, liver, gallbladder, kidney, and colon.

The important bottom line is that based on virtually all the scientific evidence discovered around the world, excess body weight in the form of fat is generally recognized to increase the risks for chronic diseases.

MEDICAL MEASURE OF BODY WEIGHT
The most common available means of classifying weight in medicine is the Body Mass Index, or BMI. This is a mathematical calculation, using both a person's height and weight, because it stands to reason that a shorter person should carry less weight than a taller person. The number produced by using both parameters is the BMI of the individual, and indicates whether the person's weight is normal, overweight, or obese. Being overweight increases many risks for unhealthful disorders and being

obese increases these risks even more. Further on in this chapter, charts are provided to help you find your BMI.

If you like calculating numbers, this is the formula for adults:

Weight in kilos / height in meters squared or kg/m^2

For example, this is the calculation for a person who weighs 70 kilos (154 pounds) and is 1.75 meters (5 feet 7 inches) tall:

70 kg / (1.75 m²) = 70 / 3.06 = 22.9
BMI = 22.9

In different parts of the world, the classifications within the BMI vary. As an example, these are the North American classifications: BMI below 18.5 is underweight. BMI between 18.5 and 24.9 indicates normal weight. BMI of 25 to 29.9 is overweight and 30 and above is obese. For children, the calculations are more complex, because they also take age into account. At the end of this chapter, there are links to online BMI calculators for adults and children.

For adults, obesity is sometimes classified further:

Obese Class I: BMI 30 to 34.9
Obese Class II: BMI 35 to 39.9
Obese Class III: BMI 40 or higher

For medical purposes, the general rule is that the higher the BMI outside the "normal" range, the greater the risk for chronic disease. Suffice it to say, classifying levels of obesity helps to assess a patient's risks and eventual needs.

A word of caution: The danger from being overweight or obese arises from excess body fat accumulation and not muscle, organ, or bone weight. Why is this important? An example might give us the answer. Two people having the same scale weight may have different amounts of fat. One person may possess a lot of muscle and very little fat, but weigh the same as another with little muscle and a lot of fat. Being muscular with little body fat is not unhealthy, and the BMI method does not detect that situation, so it is not perfect. For example, using the classifications listed above makes virtually every "well-conditioned" athlete in professional football obese, according to their BMI. Nonetheless, using the BMI is a good initial way in most cases to assess overweight and obesity.

It is also important to realize that loss of muscle and bone mineral density (BMD) can be an often-overlooked, negative effect of weight loss programs. Any weight-loss program that reduces fat but also reduces muscle and BMD will lessen the benefits of the fat loss. In other words, it is not the only the amount, but also the kind of weight one loses that is the true test of safety and efficacy of a weight-loss effort. Remember, insulin resistance favors accumulation of fat coinciding with muscle loss.

Optimal weight loss is loss of body fat. When the glucose-insulin system is working as it should, it helps to maintain a healthy ratio of fat to muscle, and I will talk more about this in later chapters. The most accurate measure of fat, muscle, and organs in a human body requires special equipment in a medical setting, equipment that is not used in typical medical offices. For home use, there are scales that measure body composition as well as total weight. These are not as accurate as the medical tests but may be helpful in tracking progress when following a weight-loss program. Waist size, along with scale weight, can help to estimate the influence of a particular weight-loss regimen.

WAIST SIZE

Fat around the waist, often called "belly fat," is more dangerous than fat in other parts of the body. Belly fat suggests the presence of insulin resistance and raises risk for diabetes and heart disease even more than overall excess weight. For this reason, waist size is another indicator of health risk. Large waist sizes indicate that insulin resistance has most likely developed, and there is higher risk for diabetes and heart disease.

Different health organizations assess the exact point in waist measurements where risk increases a bit differently.

AMERICAN HEART ASSOCIATION

Women's waist: Bigger than 35 inches (88 cm)
Men's waist: Bigger than 40 inches (102 cm)

INTERNATIONAL DIABETES FEDERATION

Women's waist: Bigger than 31.5 inches (80 cm)
Men's waist: Bigger than 35.5 inches (90 cm)

A LITTLE WEIGHT LOSS HELPS A LOT

I find that people are often surprised by how much difference in overall health a little weight loss can make. The Diabetes Prevention Program I described in the previous chapter showed that losing between 5 and 7 percent of body weight prevented development of the disease in many people who were at high risk for diabetes. Other studies have found that about half of those at high risk for diabetes did not develop the disease with weight loss between 2.3 and 4.2 percent of their initial body weight. In these successful programs, a combination of diet and exercise produced the beneficial results.

How to Find BMI

For adults, there is a calculator at:
www.nhlbi.nih.gov/health/educational/lose_wt/BMI/bmicalc.htm

For children and teenagers, there is a calculator at:
https://nccd.cdc.gov/dnpabmi/Calculator.aspx

Adults can also use the charts below. On the first chart, find your height in the column on the left, and then look to the right to find your weight. The BMI will be at the top of that column. If your weight is not in the first chart, look for it in the second chart.

This is what BMI indicates:

Below 18.5: underweight
Between 18.5 and 24.9: normal weight
Between 25 and 29.9: overweight
At or above 30: obese

BMI	19	20	21	22	23	24	25	26	27	28	29	30	31	32	33	34	35
Height (inches)							Body Weight (pounds)										
58	91	96	100	105	110	115	119	124	129	134	138	143	148	153	158	162	167
59	94	99	104	109	114	119	124	128	133	138	143	148	153	158	163	168	173
60	97	102	107	112	118	123	128	133	138	143	148	153	158	163	168	174	179
61	100	106	111	116	122	127	132	137	143	148	153	158	164	169	174	180	185
62	104	109	115	120	126	131	136	142	147	153	158	164	169	175	180	186	191
63	107	113	118	124	130	135	141	146	152	158	163	169	175	180	186	191	197
64	110	116	122	128	134	140	145	151	157	163	169	174	180	186	192	197	204
65	114	120	126	132	138	144	150	156	162	168	174	180	186	192	198	204	210
66	118	124	130	136	142	148	155	161	167	173	179	186	192	198	204	210	216
67	121	127	134	140	146	153	159	166	172	178	185	191	198	204	211	217	223
68	125	131	138	144	151	158	164	171	177	184	190	197	203	210	216	223	230
69	128	135	142	149	155	162	169	176	182	189	196	203	209	216	223	230	236
70	132	139	146	153	160	167	174	181	188	195	202	209	216	222	229	236	243
71	136	143	150	157	165	172	179	186	193	200	208	215	222	229	236	243	250
72	140	147	154	162	169	177	184	191	199	206	213	221	228	235	242	250	258
73	144	151	159	166	174	182	189	197	204	212	219	227	235	242	250	257	265
74	148	155	163	171	179	186	194	202	210	218	225	233	241	249	256	264	272
75	152	160	168	176	184	192	200	208	216	224	232	240	248	256	264	272	279
76	156	164	172	180	189	197	205	213	221	230	238	246	254	263	271	279	287

Body Weight (pounds)

BMI	36	37	38	39	40	41	42	43	44	45	46	47	48	49	50	51	52	53	54
Height (inches)																			
58	172	177	181	186	191	196	201	205	210	215	220	224	229	234	239	244	248	253	258
59	178	183	188	193	198	203	208	212	217	222	227	232	237	242	247	252	257	262	267
60	184	189	194	199	204	209	215	220	225	230	235	240	245	250	255	261	266	271	276
61	190	195	201	206	211	217	222	227	232	238	243	248	254	259	264	269	275	280	285
62	196	202	207	213	218	224	229	235	240	246	251	256	262	267	273	278	284	289	295
63	203	208	214	220	225	231	237	242	248	254	259	265	270	278	282	287	293	299	304
64	209	215	221	227	232	238	244	250	256	262	267	273	279	285	291	296	302	308	314
65	216	222	228	234	240	246	252	258	264	270	276	282	288	294	300	306	312	318	324
66	223	229	235	241	247	253	260	266	272	278	284	291	297	303	309	315	322	328	334
67	230	236	242	249	255	261	268	274	280	287	293	299	306	312	319	325	331	338	344
68	236	243	249	256	262	269	276	282	289	295	302	308	315	322	328	335	341	348	354
69	243	250	257	263	270	277	284	291	297	304	311	318	324	331	338	345	351	358	365
70	250	257	264	271	278	285	292	299	306	313	320	327	334	341	348	355	362	369	376
71	257	265	272	279	286	293	301	308	315	322	329	338	343	351	358	365	372	379	386
72	265	272	279	287	294	302	309	316	324	331	338	346	353	361	368	375	383	390	397
73	272	280	288	295	302	310	318	325	333	340	348	355	363	371	378	386	393	401	408
74	280	287	295	303	311	319	326	334	342	350	358	365	373	381	389	396	404	412	420
75	287	295	303	311	319	327	335	343	351	359	367	375	383	391	399	407	415	423	431
76	295	304	312	320	328	336	344	353	361	369	377	385	394	402	410	418	426	435	443

CHAPTER 5
Poor Choices of Foods and Drinks

• • •

CONSUMING IMPROPER FOODS AND BEVERAGES can hurt the way our bodies function in many ways. What we eat and drink on a regular basis has the biggest effect. For example, drinking a soda with high sugar content once a month should not cause a problem for a healthy person, but imbibing this same amount of soda every day may contribute to insulin resistance and gain of body fat, especially if the overall diet also contains additional sources of sugar and refined carbohydrates.

It is generally recognized that the worst foods and drinks are those consumed in large quantities that cause quick, high elevations in blood glucose. As I've mentioned, such a phenomenon leads to a series of harmful changes, starting with insulin resistance and gain of body fat and progressing to diabetes, heart disease, and other medical problems. Comprehending which foods and drinks have the most dramatic, negative effects and minimizing their consumption are key steps to improving one's diet.

SUGAR IN DRINKS
Popular drinks containing sweeteners like sucrose, high fructose corn syrup, or other sweeteners listed later in this chapter are a major source

of sugar in today's diets. Studies have reported that these significantly encourage the development of insulin resistance and weight gain. In fact, convincing research reveals that in both children and adults, the trends of rising obesity and type 2 diabetes parallel the increasing popularity of sweetened drinks. How does excessive drinking of sweetened fluids bring about the associated metabolic disturbances?

When we eat nutritious solid food, our bodies recognize that we are ingesting calories as fuel, and give us signals that we are satisfied. In a healthy body, this mechanism naturally influences how much we eat and helps to control body weight. Sugar in drinks doesn't exactly work this way. Studies suggest that sweetened drinks don't completely satisfy hunger. We are likely to eat the same amount of solid food, with or without sweetened drinks. Thus, the extra calories from such drinks are more likely to be stored as fat and are a major contributor to weight gain.

Unfortunately, sodas and other sugar-loaded drinks are often consumed alone, as a snack between meals. In our digestive system, sugar is absorbed more quickly from drinks than from solid foods where there is a so-called "food effect." Consequently, sweetened drinks, especially when consumed on an empty stomach, cause a more rapid and dramatic rise in blood glucose. This is harmful; because it is more apt to create insulin resistance and diabetes. Do I have any proof of this? Studies have found that one to two sugar-sweetened drinks per day increase risk for diabetes by 26 percent. Another study found that having two sweetened drinks per day, for six months, induced some of the harmful changes that make up the metabolic syndrome, described in chapter 2. In that study, each one of the drinks contained 12 ounces, or about 470 ml.

In the past, the United States had the highest per-person consumption of drinks sweetened with sugars. However, other countries have now taken the lead. A recent analysis shows that, per person, these countries are the top five consumers of sugar-sweetened drinks:

1. Chile
2. Mexico
3. United States
4. Argentina
5. Saudi Arabia

Sweetened drinks include sodas, flavored milks, coffees, teas, fruit drinks, flavored waters, and any other type of drink with added sugar. One example would be any mixture of water, fruit, and sugar. Drinking too much pure fruit juice, even if it doesn't contain added sugar, can also cause problems.

SUGAR IN FOODS

In the United States, about three out of four packaged foods and drinks contain added sugar, and this trend has been growing around the world. Candy, sweet baked foods, and other desserts are obvious products containing sugar, but these are not the only major sources. Sugar is added to breads that we don't consider "sweet," to sauces, salad dressings, ketchup and other condiments, soups, cereals, frozen meals, yogurt, flavored cream cheese, and other foods.

Sweeteners can have different names, including:

Sugar
High fructose corn syrup
Nectar
Fruit nectar
Corn syrup

Syrup
Sorghum
Molasses
Honey
Cane sugar
Cane juice
Raw sugar
Maltose
Dextrose
Sucrose
Glucose
Fructose
Fruit juice concentrate

This is not a complete list but will give you an idea of how sweeteners might be listed as ingredients on labels of drinks and packaged foods.

THE STARCH QUANDARY

Carbohydrates are found in all plant foods, such as vegetables and grains, and thus are an important part of any diet. However, there are different types of carbohydrates and in a human body, some have a similar effect to sugar.

Carbohydrates are made of units of different sizes. Smaller units are broken down faster and absorbed more quickly, producing a faster and bigger rise in blood glucose. Bigger units take longer to be broken down and so are absorbed more slowly, producing less rise in blood glucose.

In technical terms, carbohydrates are characteristically classified by size. The smallest units are monosaccharides (single units, such as glucose) and disaccharides (two bound units, such as sucrose, composed of glucose and fructose). These smaller units are commonly referred to as sugars. Larger units consist of oligosaccharides (3-9 units) and polysaccharides (more than 10 units). Starches are made of larger units and, to be absorbed, must be broken down into smaller ones.

Compared to protein and fat, starchy foods are made up of smaller units and are absorbed more quickly, producing a fast and high rise in blood glucose, much like ordinary sugar. An important fact to remember is that even if a starchy food doesn't taste sweet, it can still act like sugar once it is digested.

Eating starchy foods in excess can contribute to insulin resistance, weight gain, and diabetes. Therefore, it is unfortunate that many packaged foods are high in both starch and added sugars. These include a lot of cereals, cakes and breads, and snack foods. Refined grains that are most often used in packaged foods contain more starch than whole, unrefined grains. White flour is a widely used refined grain.

THE GLYCEMIC INDEX

Different individual carbohydrates have been tested to see how quickly they raise blood glucose levels, and results of these tests make up the glycemic index, which is abbreviated "GI." Foods in this index are referred to as "high-GI," meaning they produce a quick, big elevation of blood glucose; "low-GI," meaning they produce a relatively slow, small rise in blood glucose; or "moderate or medium GI," with values that fall in between.

This index can be used as a guide to help choose foods and drinks that have a less dramatic effect on blood glucose and are less likely to lead to insulin resistance, weight gain, and disease – foods with a low glycemic index. Foods that contain fiber as well as starch fall in the medium or lower range of the glycemic index, because fiber slows down the absorption of sugar and starch, creating a smaller effect on blood glucose. Low-glycemic foods may also help to control appetite and fight obesity.

Meat, fish, and pure fats, such as butter or oils, are not rated on the glycemic index because they do not raise blood glucose. These are examples of how some popular carbohydrate foods rank on the index:

Low GI: Many fruits, most vegetables, legumes, chickpeas, grains that are not refined, and nuts.

Medium GI: Whole wheat, potatoes, sweet potatoes, and basmati rice.

High GI: White bread, white rice, corn flakes, and many other breakfast cereals.

The effects of sugar and starch are also influenced by other foods eaten at the same time. Fiber, fat, and protein slow down sugar and starch absorption. The effect of a combination of foods, which generally make up meals, is often referred to as the "glycemic load" of that meal. When high-glycemic foods make up only a small part of a meal, the overall glycemic load will be lower. In addition, certain dietary supplements, described in later chapters, influence sugar and starch absorption and can help to reduce the glycemic index. However, supplements are aids and do not fully replace the need to limit the amount of sugar and starch to reasonable levels in our diets.

Other than rate of absorption, the amount of the carbohydrate consumed is important. As you might expect, eating a small amount of high-glycemic food probably causes little harm, but a greater, constant consumption will most likely be harmful in the long run.

OTHER HARMFUL FOOD INGREDIENTS

Foods can contain pesticides and chemical food additives, such as colors, preservatives, and flavor enhancers. Pesticides contain toxins. In the case of food additives, some people can be sensitive to these and should avoid them, and others avoid them on principle, as there is no human nutritional need for chemical additives and some may be harmful when consumed for many years. In addition, many people are concerned about the effect of genetically modified foods, or GMOs, and some countries have laws limiting the production and importing of such foods.

Excess salt and fat can also be problematic. Most salt today comes from packaged foods and fast foods, and these should not make up most of one's diet. In the case of fat, the most harmful type is industrially produced trans fat, also called trans fatty acids. On food labels, trans fat is listed as "partially hydrogenated oil," which means an oil that has been chemically altered to become solid. Trans fats increase risks for diabetes, heart disease, and strokes.

It's also important to keep in mind that overeating in general — consuming too many calories — is not good for health. At the very least, eating too much can cause discomfort. It also leads to gain of body fat and obesity, which is part of the deadly triangle described in chapter 2. It increases risks for insulin resistance, diabetes, and heart disease.

What to Eat and Drink for Better Health

• • •

I'M NOT A PROPONENT OF highly restrictive diets because for most people, they aren't sustainable. For many years, there have been fad diets that promise quick weight loss and may work for a short time. Unfortunately, these are usually not practical long-term and eventually, most people regain weight or gain even more than they lost. I'm a big believer in making sensible dietary changes that can lead to a healthier, longer life.

The secret, as I see it, is this: Improving one's diet for better health requires making changes that become everyday eating habits. For anyone who is overweight, losing some fat weight is an important goal. For everyone, a diet that prevents or reverses insulin resistance is essential. In both cases, improvements in diet need to be realistic and practical, so that food can be enjoyed and a better way of eating becomes part of one's daily routine.

I also want to debunk an all-too-common myth. Time and again, I find people think that a healthy diet must be unpleasant, and this is simply not true. Before mass-produced foods were invented, our ancestors enjoyed plenty of flavorful, healthy dishes. Granted, they probably spent much more time preparing food, but we now have many ways to short-cut the process and still eat tasty and nutritious food. For simple ways to prepare meals, supermarkets carry plenty of pre-cut vegetables, meat, and fish that are ready to cook, as well as interesting spice blends. If you don't cook, healthy versions of take-out food are available in many supermarkets, especially ones that specialize in natural and organic food, and fast-food outlets with healthier options, such as grilled chicken and vegetables (other than French fries) are growing in popularity.

For anyone who wants to upgrade their diet, the challenge lies in identifying the most important changes that are needed, and ways to turn these into practical habits. Dietary supplements, which I'll talk about a bit later, can be a helpful aid but they aren't a substitute for sensible choices of foods and beverages. Rather than trying to give you a daily menu or lists of foods to eat or avoid, I want to look at the most important aspects of a diet that potentially help or harm well-being in the short term, and may significantly influence health and lifespan in the longer term.

CALORIES STILL COUNT

The idea of counting calories has fallen out of favor in recent years but the underlying premise — that we shouldn't eat too much — will always hold true. Regardless of where calories come from, too many of them will lead to weight gain, especially as we get older. What most people don't realize is that for anyone who is overweight, a relatively small amount of weight loss, in the form of body fat, can be beneficial. To recap an important study I described in chapter 3, a weight loss of 5 to 7 percent of initial body weight reduced risk of diabetes by an average of 58 percent, and among people age 60 and older, the risk was reduced by 71 percent.

The marketing of weight-loss diets often includes testimonials from people who lost 50 or 100 pounds, or even more. In comparison, for a 200-pound person, a loss of 10 to 14 pounds (5 to 7 percent) may not seem as dramatic, but it's much more realistic and sustainable. For anyone who is obese, I'm not suggesting that they shouldn't lose more weight but rather, I want to convey that even a smaller amount of weight loss is very worthwhile. Two things are important: The weight loss should be mostly body fat, rather than muscle, and it needs to be maintained. In other words, a heroic effort of following a fad diet for a few weeks or months, followed by weight regain, isn't the right approach. Simply eating a little less food — "portion control" is the popular phrase — is a good start, but there are a few other things to consider.

Sugars

Seven in ten Americans consume too much added sugar, meaning sugar that is not naturally present in fruit or other foods. Nearly half the added sugar comes from beverages, including sodas, fruit drinks, energy and sports drinks, and sweetened coffee and tea, with sodas accounting for over half of all sweetened drinks. Snacks and sweets make up nearly another third, and sweetened grains, such as cereals, another 8 percent.

I can't emphasize enough that sugar in drinks is especially troublesome. When we drink high-caloric, sweet beverages, they don't satisfy our appetite, and we generally eat just as much food as we would without these beverages. This produces a double insult on the glucose-insulin system. Excess sugar leads to insulin resistance, which provokes more storage of body fat, and the extra calories in sweetened drinks also lead to more body fat.

Low-calorie or no-calorie artificial sweeteners are not an effective alternative. In fact, they may make things worse by increasing appetite, contributing to insulin resistance, and promoting weight gain. One study, at Yale University, found that the intense sweetness of artificial sweeteners tricks the brain into expecting food, may contribute to increased appetite, and encourages sugar cravings and sugar dependence. Another study, at the National Institute on Aging, tracked 1,454 men and women for an average of 10 years and found that low-calorie sweeteners correlated with a heavier weight, larger waist, and more abdominal obesity, which is a sign of possible insulin resistance.

REDUCING SUGAR OVERLOAD

The US Dietary Guidelines recommend no more than 10 percent of daily calories from added sugar, which roughly translates to a daily limit of 50 grams (200 calories) or 12.5 teaspoons of added sugar. If you think about it, that's quite a lot of sugar. The American Heart Association recommends lower limits: 24 grams (100 calories) or 6 teaspoons of added sugar for women and children over age 2, 36 grams (150 calories) or 9 teaspoons for men, and no added sugar for children under the age of 2.

It's difficult to avoid overindulging in sugar while drinking sweetened beverages. One 12-ounce can of soda contains about 8 teaspoons of sugar, or 32 grams. If you routinely drink soda or other sweetened beverages, switching to something unsweetened is a major step toward avoiding health problems. Sugar essentially has an "addictive effect" and changing habits is a challenging process, but not an impossible one. Taste buds that are accustomed to very sweet drinks will need to adjust, and this can take a few weeks. But, if you give your body a chance, it will happen.

Water is a good option. To vary its taste without adding sugar, try adding some cucumber or fruit slices to a jug of water and letting it sit in the fridge for a while. The fruit flavor will be mild but refreshing. Or, squeeze a few drops of juice from an orange, lemon, or lime into a glass of water or plain sparkling water. If you like unsweetened tea or coffee, either caffeinated or decaf versions are options. Avoiding candy and other sweet snacks is another helpful step.

STARCHES

Keep in mind that starchy foods, especially refined grains, can work just like sugar in the human body and contribute to insulin resistance, and refined grain foods are also likely to contain a lot of added sugar. Refined cereals and snack foods are major sources of these. Whole grain cereals are a better choice, as long as they are low in sugar.

Whole fruit can be a replacement for starchy or sugary snacks. Although fruit naturally contains a variety of sugars – pure fructose in addition to sucrose — it also contains beneficial nutrients as well as fiber, which reduce the impact of the fruit sugar. However, fruit juices, and drinks that contain concentrated sugar without fiber, are not good options for preventing insulin resistance. Adding fiber to the diet can be as important as limiting sugar intake.

APPETITE CONTROL AND WEIGHT LOSS

Numerous studies show that limiting carbohydrates, by eating less sugar and starch, is an effective way to lose weight and improve overall health. Eating this way improves blood glucose and controls appetite more effectively than other types of diets. The best way to reduce carbohydrates is to prepare and eat fresh, whole foods and avoid breads made with refined grains. Foods that naturally contain fiber and are rich in water, such as vegetables and fruits, increase satisfaction. Whole, unrefined grains are also a source of fiber.

Vegetables deserve special mention. As well as being rich in nutrients and fiber, they are satisfying. And, both fruits and vegetables are sources of potassium, an essential mineral that helps to control blood pressure and balance sodium in processed foods. However, it's important to eat plenty on non-starchy vegetables, grilled or steamed rather than fried. If you're wondering which vegetables are starchy, think of potatoes and other root vegetables. I'm not suggesting completely avoiding these, but eat them in moderation, and focus on filling more of your plate with green and other, multicolored vegetables.

It's important to recognize that habits take time to develop and they take time to change. Short-term, difficult diets will not lead to long-term improvements in weight or health. I recommend taking some time to find satisfying substitutes for soda, other sugary drinks and foods, refined carbohydrates, and unhealthy fats such as trans fats (partially hydrogenated oils). Aim to replace one item at a time with a healthier alternative. Try out different ways to make a new choice appealing and give your taste buds a chance to experience flavors other than intense sweetness and starch. Little by little, you can take steps forward on a lasting path to better health.

Easy Ways to be More Active

• • •

MUCH LIKE A PROPER DIET, physical activity is an important component of a lifestyle designed to bring about optimal health. For many years, it has been generally accepted that exercise reduces accumulation of body fat, helps to preserve and build muscle, strengthens bones, enhances mental performance and mood, and improves overall physical function as we get older. Of utmost significance, physical activity additionally reduces the chances of developing severe forms of heart disease, diabetes, and other ills.

To give you an idea of just how powerful exercise can be, one study found that compared to physically active people, those who are not active are twice as likely to develop heart disease. In some other cases, the benefits of exercise are even more dramatic. A study of men found that improving physical fitness reduced their risk of early death from any cause by 44 percent. Among middle-aged women, the combination of a healthy diet and exercise decreased the incidence of heart disease events by 80 percent. Studies also found that exercise reduces, and sometimes even reverses insulin resistance. Remember, insulin resistance is an early step in the chain of events that leads to obesity, diabetes, and heart disease.

Two Main Types of Exercise

Exercise falls into these two main categories:

Aerobic activity: Aerobic exercise is any movement that speeds up the rate at which the heart beats, such as walking, running, or jumping. The heart is a special type of muscle, and when physical activity makes it beat faster, it is strengthening that muscle. The main job of the heart is to keep pumping blood, which delivers vital oxygen and nutrients to every part of the body. A strong heart is more efficient, doesn't work as hard to pump lots of blood, and can keep us alive and well for a lot of years.

Resistance or weight training: This is any type of exercise that makes skeletal muscles work harder and makes them stronger and, sometimes, bigger. Lifting weights falls into this category. Other types of resistance exercise may use the person's own body weight for resistance. Push-ups, sit-ups, and squats are examples of resistance exercises that don't require weights.

Both types of exercise may increase insulin sensitivity. In other words, they help to prevent, improve, and/or reverse insulin resistance. In turn, enhancing insulin sensitivity reduces the risks for weight gain, diabetes, and heart disease. Both types, aerobic and resistance training, are also helpful for weight loss and, after losing weight, for preventing weight regain. For anyone who doesn't exercise regularly, it's understandable that trying to start different types of exercise at the same time may be difficult. I like to take a realistic view and recommend starting by walking.

The Benefits of Walking

I believe walking is the foundation of a good exercise program for people of all ages, especially for those who are not athletically inclined. It's therapeutic, doesn't require any special skills or equipment, and can be carried out almost anywhere, anytime. Research supports this view, showing that walking is an effective first step toward improved fitness and health. Walking can be done by one individual alone, or with a group, making it somewhat of a social activity. In fact, studies have found that among older people, walking is the most popular type of activity and has a very low risk of injury. In addition, older adults are more likely to continue a walking program than other, more strenuous types of physical activity.

Research has shown that regular moderate exercise, such as walking, significantly reduces the incidence of diabetes. More specifically, a review of 23 studies, with a total of more than 1.2 million people, found that the equivalent of walking 30 minutes daily, on 5 days per week, reduced risk of diabetes by 26 percent. Additional exercise, either for longer periods of time and/or with more intense activity, reduced risk even further.

Helpful Tools

There are many gadgets today that track physical activity, such as apps in smartphones or fitness trackers worn on the wrist, and these can be helpful. Personally, I recommend using a very simple and inexpensive tool, a pedometer. It clips on to a belt or other clothing and counts the number of steps a person takes. Pedometers are small and light, can easily be worn throughout the day, and will continually measure steps a person takes. Simply set the counter to zero at the beginning of the day and see how many steps you've taken as the day progresses.

To increase physical activity, it's important to set goals and measure progress. A pedometer can help you do that and can motivate you to move more. A daily total of 10,000 steps is usually recommended. However, adding about 3,000 steps to your usual daily total has also been shown to be therapeutic, especially if you walk at a pace of about 100 steps per minute. This speed is considered "brisk walking."

Tracking steps taken each day has been shown to be an effective tool to increase physical activity. A review of 26 studies, with a total of more than 2,700 people, found that using a pedometer was associated with an increase of 2,000 steps per day, which led to some weight loss and a significant reduction in blood pressure. Another study tested a walking program with a pedometer for weight loss, among 307 people. Without changing diet, those in the program increased their daily activity by the equivalent of walking an extra mile per day and lost almost 3 pounds during 4 weeks.

PLANNING

Many people like to walk in the morning, before they start their day, but a walk can be beneficial at any time. For people with type 2 diabetes, one study found that taking a walk after meals, especially meals with carbohydrates, was most effective at controlling levels of blood glucose.

As a rule, try to walk 30 minutes at a brisk pace on at least five days of the week. If 30 minutes is too difficult to work in to your schedule, aim for shorter walks of at least 10 minutes each. Other forms of exercise that increase your heart rate are equally beneficial, and include dancing or playing any sport. Once you have a walking routine, consider adding some form of resistance exercise. To learn movements, try a group class or video workouts, online or on DVDs. It's also important to find activities that you enjoy, as it's more likely that you will continue to do these.

To summarize, each of us is unique, and only you know what you like. Some people prefer to walk alone while others enjoy getting together for a walk with friends or family. And, 30 minutes a day is not a limit but a minimum, as more exercise generally produces more benefits. The most important thing is to make walking and other forms of physical activity a regular part of your life.

CHAPTER 8

Dietary Supplements: Aids in Prevention

• • •

WHILE LIFESTYLE CHANGES THAT PREVENT insulin resistance are essential for better health, I also believe that dietary supplements offer additional, complementary benefits. Combined with a proper diet and exercise regimen, supplements can provide safe ways to help achieve health goals faster and more completely. In contrast, I cannot recommend chronic use of current anti-diabetic drugs for prevention.

Although medicinal drugs that treat type 2 diabetes are sometimes suggested as means to prevent chronic glucose-insulin disturbances and diabetes, I feel they, on many occasions, are not as practical or safe as a healthy lifestyle, alone or in combination with natural dietary supplements. Experience suggests that drugs may help prevent some cases of diabetes, but only as long as they are taken on a continual basis, and this is associated with the development of many unintended risks.

Continual use of natural dietary supplements for prevention offers a better way to enhance the beneficial effects of diet and exercise over the long haul. As a general rule, natural supplements are typically less potent than drugs but don't usually cause the same deleterious side effects. A boon to most dietary regimens, supplements are also relatively inexpensive. For these reasons, in contrast to drugs, I consider some natural dietary supplements to be a practical, safe aid for prevention.

Nevertheless, there are countless people who suffer from the ravages of type 2 diabetes and require prescription drugs to survive in a reasonable fashion. This brings on a dilemma. In the case of the treatment for diabetes and even obesity, prescription medicines have a strong history of serious adverse side effects, particularly cardiovascular events. These can be especially injurious when the drugs are taken for many years. As a result, new drugs are continually being produced.

Drugs that treat type 2 diabetes work to lower levels of blood glucose in a few different ways (some natural supplements work in similar ways, but are more gentle). These include stimulating more production or release of insulin, increasing sensitivity to insulin, or blocking the absorption of carbohydrates. Depending on the drug, side effects may include digestive upset, weight gain, swelling due to fluid retention, liver problems, heart problems, hypoglycemia (blood glucose that is dangerously low), and lactic acidosis (too much lactic acid).

In healthy people, lactic acid is a substance that accumulates in muscles as a result of strenuous exercise. The presence of lactic acid is one reason why muscles get sore from exercise. Among people taking certain diabetes drugs, lactic acid can accumulate in the blood. It can be quite dangerous and requires medical attention. These are some symptoms of lactic acidosis:

Stomach upset
Diarrhea
Loss of appetite
Muscle cramps
Feeling sleepy or tired
Weakness

DANGERS OF LOW BLOOD GLUCOSE

Diabetes drugs, especially those that stimulate production of insulin, can lower blood glucose too much. Blood-glucose levels that are too low, called "hypoglycemia", can be dangerous and can cause a variety of symptoms, including these:

Feeling shaky or jittery
Sweating
Hunger
Headache
Blurred vision
Feeling sleepy or tired
During sleep, crying out or having nightmares
Becoming dizzy or lightheaded
Feeling confused or disoriented
Becoming pale
Being uncoordinated
Getting irritable or nervous
Being argumentative or combative

Having trouble concentrating
Becoming weak
Having a fast or irregular heart beat
Loss of appetite
Changes in behavior or personality

Severely low concentrations of blood glucose are associated with sei-zures, convulsions, or unconsciousness. Because of the possibility of hypoglycemia, this is one time when I advise patients to carry around some form of sugar, even a candy bar. Remember, it's only for an emergency.

DIETARY SUPPLEMENTS

Keep in mind that by far the most common disturbance in the human glucose-insulin system begins with insulin resistance -- not a lack of insu-lin. Cells in muscles and other parts of the body are not able to absorb blood glucose, so circulating glucose levels in the blood become elevat-ed. Fortunately, this problem can often be reversed with natural dietary supplements, so-called "insulin sensitizers" -- meaning they increase the body's natural sensitivity to insulin. Chromium, an essential mineral that I discuss in the next chapter, is one of my top choices. It helps reduce blood glucose when it is too high but does not lower it below healthy levels. Very importantly, natural insulin sensitizers can reduce injurious circulat-ing insulin levels when these are too high.

Some herbs can stimulate more production and release of insulin. Although they are not as strong as drugs, they may work through a simi-lar mechanism. I don't recommend these types of supplements, because they don't solve the real problem of insulin resistance, and may cause levels of blood glucose to drop too low. In addition, high levels of insulin produce many of the harmful effects associated with diabetes.

Supplements that slow and reduce absorption of sugar and starch are other practical aids to safely lower blood glucose, and can also help prevent weight gain and assist with weight loss. Because of their mechanisms of action, these supplements are commonly referred to as "carb blockers" and include a white bean extract, hibiscus extract, and l-arabinose.

To combat the bitter sweet, "bitter herbs" can afford some benefits.

Since weight gain is a big part of the blood-glucose problem, a natural supplement that helps to burn fat, bitter orange, is another useful aid. In addition, bitter melon helps to reduce blood glucose and improves other aspects of health. All these supplements can work, to some extent, through different mechanisms and are described in more detail in the next few chapters.

Improving Insulin Sensitivity with Chromium

• • •

AVOIDING TOO MUCH DIETARY SUGAR is a good way to prevent or reduce insulin resistance and improve health, but this is a difficult task for most people. Natural dietary supplements that make cells more sensitive to insulin — insulin sensitizers — can help to reduce damage from the effects of excess dietary sugar. Chromium, an essential mineral found in very small amounts in food, is one of the most important insulin-sensitizing supplements we can take to help overcome several serious maladies, including obesity, type 2 diabetes, elevated blood pressure, high triglycerides, low "good" HDL-cholesterol, and persistent inflammation.

It's important to note that there are different forms of chromium. Sometimes, this leads to confusion and unnecessary concern about the safety of chromium supplements. When I talk about the benefits of chromium, I am referring to "trivalent" chromium. This form is an essential nutrient required for sugar and fat metabolism, and is added to foods and supplements for purposes of enhancing health. In contrast, another form — "hexavalent" chromium —is generally known to be toxic. Don't worry: this form of the element is not used in supplements. Studies described later in this chapter, and my discussion and recommendations all refer to the safe, non-toxic, trivalent form of chromium.

Both my wife and I have been taking chromium on a daily basis for over 20 years, and I'm convinced it has helped us stay in optimal health and live very active lives. Both of us could have retired early, but we chose to continue working full-time in demanding careers, for love of our occupations. Although chromium is not a substitute for reducing sugar consumption and eating a healthy diet, it is a valuable aid.

CAN FOOD PROVIDE ENOUGH CHROMIUM?

There is much controversy over the daily amount of chromium needed for optimal health. In the United States, the National Academy of Sciences' Food and Nutrition Board has set an estimated safe and adequate daily dietary intake (ESADDI) of chromium. The amount is measured in micrograms. To put quantities in context, 1 gram contains 1,000 milligrams, abbreviated as mg, and 1 milligram contains 1,000 micrograms, abbreviated as mcg.

The ESADDI is 50-200 mcg per day. Despite this seemingly low intake, the average amount of chromium people consume is generally even lower, much less than the minimum 50 mcg per day. This is not optimal at any age, and chromium concentrations in the human body decrease significantly as we get older. This is unfortunate, because cells naturally become less sensitive to insulin later in life and lack of chromium can only make matters worse.

Although food is generally considered the best source of nutrients, this is an unrealistic notion in the case of chromium. (See some examples of chromium amounts in food, later in this chapter.) Even a well-balanced meal plan designed by the most skilled of nutritionists cannot provide the minimum ESADDI of 50 mcg per day. Dr. Richard Anderson, an expert in the field, estimates that to meet minimal requirements from diet alone, an individual would have to consume from 3,000 to 10,000 calories, amounts that could lead to extreme obesity. In addition, common stresses can alter chromium metabolism and increase the amount an individual requires. Such stresses include consuming a large amount of sugar at one time, continually eating a diet high in sugars and starches, breast-feeding, infection, strenuous exercise, and physical trauma. In short, it is virtually impossible to get enough chromium from food alone.

How Chromium Works

Chromium is essential for healthy digestion of sugar, as well as other types of food. Chromium makes cells more sensitive to insulin, enabling blood glucose to be taken in by cells and used throughout the body to make energy. Ironically, the risk of a chromium deficiency is especially high when we consume large amounts of sugar and refined carbohydrates, because a high-sugar diet causes the human body to excrete more of the mineral.

The action of chromium began to be recognized by scientists in the mid-1950s, -- principally from animal studies. The connection between the mineral and human health began to be observed about 20 years later, when patients who were being fed intravenously mysteriously developed signs of diabetes. The intravenous feeding fluid did not contain chromium, and the patients subsequently developed a deficiency. When chromium was added to the intravenous formula, the diabetes symptoms disappeared.

Since then, numerous studies have demonstrated that chromium supplements can produce healthier levels of blood glucose and insulin.

Research from various laboratories has also shown that lowering blood glucose helps to bring blood pressure and cholesterol into healthier ranges.

As an example, a study of 180 men and women with type 2 diabetes tested two doses of chromium supplements: 100 mcg or 500 mcg, taken twice daily, for a total of 200 mcg or 1,000 mcg per day. Blood glucose levels were much improved in those taking 1,000 mcg after two months, and after four months for those taking 200 mcg. Insulin levels began to improve with both dosages after two months. Among those taking 1,000 mcg daily, cholesterol levels also improved after four months.

Studies have also tested chromium taken in addition to diabetes drugs, and found that adding the mineral improved levels of blood glucose, more than drugs alone. In addition, people taking the chromium gained less weight than those taking only the drugs. I believe that over the long term, chromium could help to prevent many cases of diabetes and improve treatment in other settings without the undesired side effects of drugs.

Several studies have found, when assessing weight loss regimens, that along with a program of diet and/or exercise, added chromium can be helpful. Even more importantly, chromium can bring about more "proper" weight loss. Let me explain that further.

In one study, where I was one of the researchers, we found that addition of chromium in the face of caloric restriction, compared to caloric restriction alone, did not significantly change the amount of total scale weight lost. Does this indicate that chromium had no effect? No. Further examination revealed it significantly increased fat loss in the face of decreased muscle loss — a balance that accounted for the lack of scale weight change. How does chromium accomplish this? High blood glucose concentrations are associated with high levels of circulating insulin (insulin resistance), and high insulin leads to more accumulation of body fat and muscle loss. Chromium, as an insulin sensitizer, provides the remedy by lowering insulin concentrations.

The sparing or even gain of muscle is important for optimal health in a so-called weight reduction program, and is the reason behind my reference to "proper" weight loss. Any diet that reduces the total amount of calories consumed will produce some weight loss, but much of it will be lost muscle. Losing muscle means a slower metabolism, which makes it difficult to keep weight off and reduces strength and energy. By helping to preserve muscle while making it easier for the human body to reduce fat mass, chromium can help to keep the proper weight off in the future. I tell anyone who is trying to lose weight to take chromium. It isn't a magic weight-loss pill but if taken regularly, over time, it can make a significant improvement in body composition.

One word of warning — ironically, using chromium and other insulin sensitizers can produce a bittersweet outcome in our pursuit to "lose weight." The sweet outcome, of course, is sparing or even gain in muscle mass. Now for the bitter outcome which, in truth, is really not bitter at all. Because of the widespread problem of obesity, most individuals are "addicted" to their bathroom scales. This small device gets a continual, daily use or abuse by many; and to most users, the changes in scale weight are monitored without much thought to fat loss or fat gain — only changes in total weight. Obviously, if chromium spares or even brings about a gain in muscle, the loss of fat can be obscured when examining the scale.

I have seen many a subject in research studies be misguided by bathroom scales. This is what sometimes happens in a study where some people are given a placebo and others are given a chromium supplement, but they don't know which one they are taking. If the scale weight doesn't change appreciably, many mistakenly believe they are taking the placebo, and stop following the regimen. I've had women tell me, "My weight is not changing," and a couple of minutes later, add, "but my dress size is getting smaller." Men might declare, "but my belt is looser."

What could be happening that's causing confusion? The loss of fat can be hidden by a gain in muscle, a phenomenon not unusual for chromium takers (and a good thing). Muscle is denser and heavier than fat, so a pound of muscle occupies less space than a pound of fat. As an analogy, compare the weight and size of a feather pillow and a brick. The pillow is much larger than the brick, but lighter. I'm not saying that fat is as light as a feather, but want to convey the general idea. It is possible to lose the same weight of fat as the weight of muscle gained, to account for little change in scale weight but a slimming down.

The truth is that when you lose fat and gain muscle, you become healthier, but the scale may not show the progress. Who is better off — the patient lauded by his physician for losing six pounds of weight (three pounds of fat loss and three pounds of muscle loss), or the patient derided by his doc for losing no poundage, when in fact that patient lost three pounds of fat and gained three pounds of muscle? I will take the latter result any time. Think about it: Three pounds of lost fat removes more bulk than three pounds added by muscle, so it produces a slimmer appearance. It also improves strength and enhances insulin sensitivity. An individual whose weight loss is primarily in the form of muscle has not done himself well. To me, changes in body composition are much more important than those in body weight.

Chapter 9

CHROMIUM AND AGING

Our sensitivity to insulin characteristically decreases as we get older. Although not every older person will develop insulin resistance to a harmful degree, many will, because of today's diets and inactive lifestyles. My research and other studies have shown that chromium can help us to stay healthy in several ways as we age.

Insulin resistance is the internal mechanism that leads to bigger waists and bigger bellies that we often see our friends and relatives develop with the aging process. In turn, excess fat around one's middle makes the human body even more insulin resistant, beginning a vicious cycle. With age, we also lose muscle, which makes us weaker, less likely to be physically active, and more likely to gain excess body fat.

All these changes lead to the ailments that become more common with age, including type 2 diabetes, heart disease, weight gain, high blood pressure, high cholesterol, cataracts, and inflammatory diseases which can affect joints and various organs. Interestingly, the same types of changes are also seen when there is a deficiency of chromium.

The aging process is difficult to study in people, because such clinical studies would have to last many decades. It is much more practical to study in animals, who have a much shorter lifespan. My studies, as well as those of others, have suggested that insulin resistance is a basic, internal mechanism that leads to premature aging. In one of my animal studies, chromium helped to reverse insulin resistance and extend life by up to 20 percent.

PREVENTION IS THE BEST APPROACH!

From all the scientific information gathered so far, it seems that preventing and reversing insulin resistance can be very important for anyone who wants to live a longer life and should certainly improve health at all stages, especially as we get older. I believe that chromium supplements, taken daily, can help to keep blood glucose and insulin in healthy ranges and stop or reduce insulin resistance and the harm it causes.

People who are most likely to lack sufficient chromium include:

- Anyone who consumes sweetened sodas or other sweetened drinks or foods
- Anyone who regularly eats foods made with refined grains, such as white breads, white rice, noodles, tortillas, buns, cakes, pretzels, and other starchy foods and snacks
- The elderly
- Women who are breast feeding
- Athletes or people who do a lot of physical exercise
- Anyone who has recently experienced an injury or physical trauma, or has an infection
- Anyone taking antacids, corticosteroids, or heartburn drugs

HOW TO GET ENOUGH CHROMIUM

To prevent or reverse insulin resistance, I recommend getting at least 200 mcg per day for most healthy people. Where elevated blood glucose is a problem, higher amounts may be needed. Chromium in food is not highly bioactive, meaning it isn't readily absorbed, and amounts of the mineral in food are quite small. Here are some examples of healthy foods that provide chromium:

½ cup broccoli: 11 mcg
3 ounces lean beef or turkey breast: 2 mcg
½ cup green beans: 1 mcg
1 medium apple: 1 mcg
1 medium banana: 1 mcg

As you can see, obtaining 200 mcg daily from food would be an impossible task. Supplements are a simple way to get an adequate amount, but not all chromium supplements are equally effective, as some forms are absorbed better than others.

I personally use a form called chromium polynicotinate. The chromium is bound with vitamin B3, also called niacin or nicotinic acid. This form of the supplement is also called niacin-bound chromium. Studies have shown that it is well absorbed and produces good results in lowering blood glucose and insulin. Other absorbable, or bioactive forms, are chromium picolinate and chromium histidinate.

Where blood glucose and insulin are in a healthy range, the chromium will help to keep them there, and will not drive levels too low or produce side effects. Where levels are elevated, improvements from chromium will usually be detected in less than one month. Changes in triglycerides and cholesterol may take several months. Chromium supplements are safe, as found in many studies, and have not produced adverse effects.

For anyone who is taking drugs to treat diabetes and wants to try chromium, it's important to check blood glucose regularly and work with a health professional who understands the effects of chromium. It's possible that the dose for medications already being received may need to be adjusted, or that chromium may help to reverse the condition. However, individual situations vary and it's important to do what is most beneficial for you.

For weight loss, chromium works best with a diet that contains fewer calories than you normally consume, but it doesn't have to be extreme, and adding exercise will produce even better results. The chromium will increase the amount of fat lost and help to preserve muscle. The most important thing to understand is that chromium does not create sudden weight loss. It improves the internal processes that lead to fat loss. Combining it with other, complementary supplements can enhance the overall benefits.

Other natural dietary supplements that I have studied and found safe and effective in sensitizing the activity of insulin and decreasing elevated systolic blood pressure are:

Maitake mushroom, fraction SX
Cinnamon
Bitter melon
Astaxanthin

CHAPTER 10
Supplements that Block Sugar and Starch Absorption

• • •

NATURAL DIETARY SUPPLEMENTS REFERRED TO as "carb blockers" improve glucose-insulin metabolism through an entirely different mechanism than insulin sensitizers such as chromium. How do they work? They block a goodly portion of the intestinal absorption of sucrose and starches, both slowing absorption (thus lowering the glycemic index) and reducing the number of calories ingested. This is tantamount to limiting the amount of sugar and refined starches in the diet. You might remember that starch in refined carbohydrates can act like sugar in the human body, and when eaten in excess, contributes to unhealthy, elevated levels of blood glucose, weight gain, and other ills.

Many people have had some success in losing weight with low-carb diets, which severely reduce or eliminate sugary and starchy foods. However, such diets are also difficult to sustain and many dieters regain weight, and sometimes become even heavier than they were before the diet. Carb blocker supplements can help like low-carb diets, but with less severe restriction of foods. There are at least two different mechanisms to inhibit absorption, one primarily for starch and another primarily for sugar, but there can be an overlap — the same substance may block both sugar and starches.

THE PROBLEM WITH STARCH

Starch is a natural part of many foods. Most foods that come from plants contain some starch, including beans, grains, and many vegetables and fruits. Therefore, I am not suggesting that we should avoid all starch. All these categories of food provide nutrients and can be part of a healthy diet, with one caution: Refined grains are higher in starch than whole grains and contain fewer nutrients. Although it isn't practical for most people to exclude all refined grains, they should not be eaten in too large quantities.

Starches become a problem when we eat too much of them, which is easy to do. Inexpensive, high-starch foods are all around us. Sandwiches are made with big rolls or buns. Starchy snack foods, such as cakes, cookies, and pretzels are everywhere. Different cuisines have their own types of bread or bread-like foods, such as tortillas, naan, or pita, and various types of pasta and noodles are popular around the world. Most of these are made with refined grain.

Potatoes are another major source of excess starch, in French fries and many varieties of chips, which are easy to reach for as a snack. Obviously, some of these snacks are also high in fat calories, which poses a further major challenge to most dieters. White rice, also high in starch, is a staple in various cuisines and most nutritionists favor a switch to less refined brown rice.

HOW SUPPLEMENTS BLOCK STARCH

When we digest foods, enzymes in our bodies break down the larger carbohydrate components into smaller units so that we can absorb nutrients and eliminate waste. Only the smallest sugar units (a single sugar unit is referred to as a monosaccharide) can be absorbed. Different enzymes split apart different components of food. Starch is broken down by an enzyme called amylase, released into saliva by salivary glands and into the small intestines by the pancreas. Supplements that block starch inhibit the amylase enzyme and as a result, some of the starch is not broken down. Consequently, the supplements slow down starch absorption, lowering the food's glycemic index, described in chapter 5. The overall effect is the same as eating less starch.

What happens to the unabsorbed food? In the digestive system, it moves into the large bowel, where it is fermented by bacteria. This process is both good and bad. On the good side, many of the resulting fermented products are recognized for improving our overall health. On the bad side, the fermented products, especially in the form of gases, can lead to gastrointestinal distress such as cramps.

Taking a starch-blocking supplement doesn't mean you can eat giant portions of starchy foods. Although it allows for some leeway, dietary restriction is still important to gain maximal benefits. Thus, starch-blocking supplements can augment the amount of weight loss. They can also help maintain a lower weight after a successful dietary regimen. This is very important, as practically everyone recognizes the troubling fact that it's harder to maintain a lower weight than it is to lose weight in the first place.

For optimal benefit, it's best to take carb-blocking supplements before a meal and eat a moderate amount of starchy food. When I take my family out to an Italian restaurant and we're going to eat pasta, I frequently give the supplements to everybody and we take them before our meal.

RESEARCH RESULTS

Probably, the most widely researched starch blocker is a white bean extract called Phase 2, and I am one of a number of researchers who have investigated it. Altogether, there have been at least 16 studies of Phase 2, and I wrote a chapter about it for a medical textbook. The research has shown a significant benefit of greater weight loss among people on a diet. Equally important, the supplement reduces the rise of blood glucose after starchy meals, which can help to reduce risks for diabetes, high blood pressure, and heart disease. The studies have also found that Phase 2 is safe and rarely causes significant side effects.

Research at the University of Scranton in Pennsylvania found that Phase 2 reduced starch absorption between 28 and 66 percent. The difference depended on the dose of the supplement and the contents of a meal. When high-starch food, such as white bread, is eaten alone, it raises blood sugar more quickly and dramatically than white bread plus foods that contain fiber, fat, or protein, which slow absorption. In the study, the biggest effect of Phase 2 supplements occurred when people ate white bread by itself.

One of the studies I co-authored tested Phase 2 for weight loss among 60 people in Italy. Those in the study were between the ages of 20 and 45 and were between 5 kg (11 lbs) and 15 kg (33 lbs) overweight. Their weight had not changed during the previous six months. During the study, they ate a diet that contained 2,000 to 2,200 calories per day, which is considered an average amount by American standards. Although this was not designed to be a reduced-calorie diet, many people do eat more on a regular basis. Each day, one meal contained most of the starchy foods. Before that meal, half the people in the study took 450 mg of a Phase 2 supplement and the other half took a dummy pill. None of them reported any major unpleasant side effects. After 30 days of following the program, these were the differences in average results:

Weight loss
Phase 2 supplement: 2.94 kg (6.45 lbs)
Dummy pill: 0.35 kg (0.77 lbs)

Loss of body fat
Phase 2 supplement: 10.45%
Dummy pill: 0.16%

Smaller waist size
Phase 2 supplement: 2.93 cm
Dummy pill: 0.46 cm

Smaller hip size
Phase 2 supplement: 1.48 cm
Dummy pill: 0.11 cm

Another study I co-authored tested Phase 2 on 101 healthy but overweight men and women in China, and found that the supplement can also produce weight loss without any special diet. The people in this study were between the ages of 20 and 50 and were not given any instructions about what or how much to eat. They were instructed to take 1,000 mg of the Phase 2 supplement or dummy pills three times per day, 15 minutes before each meal, for 60 days. Those taking Phase 2 lost an average of 1.9 kg (4.2 lbs) and their waist size decreased by 1.9 cm. Those taking dummy pills lost only 0.4 kg (0.9 lbs) and 0.4 cm around the waist.

Other studies found similar results in the United States and Germany, where people also reported having fewer cravings for sweet foods. When researchers in California analyzed ten earlier studies, with a total of nearly 500 people, they found that in every one, people taking Phase 2 lost significantly more weight than those taking a dummy pill. The length of these studies ranged from 4 to 12 weeks and none of them used a very restrictive diet.

All these studies show that Phase 2 is effective at reducing absorption of starchy foods and aiding with weight loss. After weight loss, it also helps to prevent weight regain. In addition, my own research with animals has found that this particular supplement also blocks some absorption of sugar.

Studies with animals have found that hibiscus extract is another natural supplement that inhibits starch absorption. It works the same way as Phase 2, by inhibiting the amylase enzyme that breaks down starch. It can be combined with Phase 2 and other helpful ingredients to reduce levels of blood glucose and help achieve or maintain a healthy weight.

How Sugar Is Blocked

When we eat or drink regular table sugar, also called sucrose, an enzyme called sucrase, located in the wall of the intestines, breaks it down into glucose and fructose so that it can be digested and absorbed. As it is absorbed, levels of blood glucose quickly rise. Consequently, eating too much sugar can lead to harmful levels. A supplement called l-arabinose inhibits the sucrase enzyme so that some of the sugar we eat cannot be broken down. The undigested sugar becomes fermented in the large bowels and much of it can be eliminated. L-arabinose doesn't block all sugar, but it does block a significant amount, so the effect is similar to eating less sugar.

STUDIES OF L-ARABINOSE

L-arabinose is a substance that is naturally present in the cell walls of some plants but it needs to be extracted and made into a supplement to reach a workable dose. My own animal research has shown that l-arabinose effectively blocks absorption of sucrose, reducing the rise in blood glucose after sweet drinks or foods are consumed. A number of other animal studies have found similar results.

The supplement has also been investigated in human studies in Japan and Denmark. In Japan, it was tested in 48 healthy people and 10 people with type 2 diabetes. In both groups, l-arabinose kept levels of blood glucose at lower levels after a sugar drink or sugar jelly. In Denmark, 15 healthy men were given sugar water on an empty stomach in the morning, a situation where blood glucose will rise very quickly and dramatically. L-arabinose significantly reduced levels of both blood glucose and insulin, which is very beneficial for overall health.

A WORD OF CAUTION

As pointed out earlier, regular sugar — sucrose — is made of two components, glucose and fructose, which are bound together. The sucrase enzyme breaks these apart and each component is then digested along a separate path in the human body. However, the two unbound simple sugars in high fructose corn syrup, which is found in many sweetened drinks and many foods, cannot be blocked, because the sucrase enzyme is not needed for separation. Like sucrose, high fructose corn syrup is made up of glucose and fructose, but they are not bound together. When we eat the corn sweetener, both components are automatically absorbed, without needing help from the sucrase enzyme. Because of this, l-arabinose will not block absorption of high fructose corn syrup.

All the supplement ingredients that block starch and sugar may be combined for best effect. In my research with animals, for example, the Phase 2 starch blocker and the l-arabinose sugar blocker worked very well together, keeping levels of blood glucose at healthier concentrations and lowering blood pressure. It is best to take them about 15-30 minutes before eating starchy and sugary food. However, they can also be effective when taken with the meal.

CHAPTER 11
Fat Burners and Other Aids

• • •

Supplements that burn fat can't replace a healthy diet and exercise but in conjunction with these, fat burners can be an aid that helps with weight loss. Keep in mind that as an additional benefit, even a little weight loss could help to reduce insulin resistance and the risk for diabetes and other health problems.

At this point, I feel obliged to digress briefly. "Fat burners" is a colorful description that "cuts to the chase." I am really talking about substances that preferentially favor the metabolism, or more simply the breakdown of fat to produce energy rather than having it accumulate into a stored lump. Bitter orange extract, also called Seville orange extract or Citrus *aurantium*, is a good fat burner that works in two ways: It helps to break down fat, and it slightly increases the number of calories used for energy by the human body.

The amount of calories a person burns is commonly referred to as their metabolic rate. If you've ever wondered why some people never seem to gain weight, no matter how much they eat, it's probably because they have a higher metabolic rate -- meaning their bodies naturally burn more calories than average. Although very few people fall into this category, these individuals do exist.

CALORIE BURNING BASICS

Even if we exercise regularly or have a physically demanding job, most of the calories we burn every day are used just to keep our bodies alive. These calories provide fuel for the heart and other functioning organs, keep blood flowing, enable us to keep breathing, and replace or repair various cells in our bodies. That process goes on around the clock, while we're awake and asleep.

Studies show that the brain, liver, heart, and kidneys, which together make up less than six percent of total body weight, burn about 60 percent of an adult's total daily calories. Skeletal muscles use between 18 and 25 percent. Skeletal muscles are attached to our bones and we use them to move our arms, legs, head, and other parts of our bodies. Internal muscles that are not under conscious control, for example, those that contract and relax the stomach, intestines, blood vessels, and bladder, burn some additional calories.

The calories required to keep us alive, even if we do nothing all day, make up what we call the resting metabolic rate. We burn additional calories as we do different types of physical activity, which includes taking a shower, brushing our teeth, walking around, and doing any type of exercise. As a rule, the fat in our bodies burns fewer calories than muscle, so people who are more muscular likely have a higher metabolic rate. Age also plays a part. Metabolic rate typically starts slowing down a bit after age 20.

"I can't eat like I used to." If you are middle-aged or older, you've probably said or thought exactly that. If you're younger, I'm sure you've heard older people say the same thing. A slower metabolic rate is one reason for changes in how much food we can eat, and it contributes to an expanding waist. One study estimated that after age 20, the total number of calories burned decreases each decade by about 150 calories per day. This may not sound like much but it means that if you eat exactly the same amount of food as you get older, you will slowly gain weight, and that's what happens to most people. Regular exercise, including some weight training to preserve and maybe build some muscle, could reduce this effect, but most people get less active as they get older.

How Bitter Orange Extract Works

Bitter orange and all other citrus fruits contain very small amounts of a natural stimulant called p-synephrine. When we eat the fruit, the amounts are, as a rule, too small to make any noticeable difference, but in concentrated extracts of bitter orange, the p-synephrine can have an important effect on fat breakdown and metabolic rate.

There are synthetic forms of this class of substances that can speed up heart rate and raise blood pressure, but the natural version in citrus fruit doesn't have these harmful effects. I and other researchers have tested bitter orange extract on people and measured heart rate, blood pressure, and other signs of possible harmful effects and have found that the natural p-synephrine in bitter orange, in amounts usually found in dietary supplements, does not cause harmful or unpleasant symptoms. However, it does provide a benefit by slightly increasing metabolic rate.

In one study I did with some of my colleagues in other research centers, different compositions and strengths of bitter orange extracts were tested. We found that metabolic rate increased between 65 and 183 calories, depending on the extract. We also reviewed more than 20 studies that tested bitter orange extract on about 360 people. These also found that the supplement was safe, increased metabolic rate, and enhanced weight loss in programs that lasted between 6 and 12 weeks.

Bitter orange extract can be taken alone but it may be even more beneficial in combination with other supplements that help to regulate blood glucose and protect against or reverse insulin resistance. Health wise, each one works in a different way to help achieve the overall goal.

BITTER MELON: ANOTHER BENEFICIAL AID

A fruit that grows in tropical parts of the world, including India, Pakistan, China, Central and South America, and East Africa, bitter melon is also called Momordica *charantia* or karela. In its native regions, it has been consumed as food and medicine for centuries. As medicine, it has been used for a variety of ailments, especially to prevent and treat obesity and diabetes.

In the past few decades, studies have found that it lowers unhealthy levels of blood glucose and provides some additional benefits. Its complete chemical composition is still being investigated but so far, it appears that a number of different ingredients found naturally in the plant work together to improve health, by regulating blood glucose and possibly other internal processes that predispose people to diabetes and heart disease.

HOW IT WORKS

Studies with healthy and diabetic animals in my lab have shown that bitter melon clears excess levels of glucose from the blood, but does not suppress levels too low. This is quite different from diabetes drugs, which can drive blood glucose below a healthy level. In addition, some bitter melon extracts, but not all, can facilitate lowering of blood pressure.

Other research with animals has found similar effects on blood glucose and other benefits. The supplement has helped to reduce insulin resistance, cholesterol, and body weight in rats. Another animal study found that bitter melon suppressed fat storage in the belly area, which is especially harmful, and reduced expansion of fat cells.

RESEARCH RESULTS

In studies of people, bitter melon has reduced unhealthy levels of blood glucose in most cases. The research methods and types of bitter melon supplements that were tested have not been consistent, and not all extracts work equally well. However, effective supplements have sometimes acted in a manner similar to diabetes drugs, without the same side effects, and sometimes with additional benefits.

One study compared the effects of two different doses of bitter melon and a diabetes drug (glibenclamide) among 95 people with type 2 diabetes. Bitter melon worked almost as well as the drug, but those taking the supplement also experienced less damage in their blood vessels, lower blood pressure, lower cholesterol, and some weight loss. In contrast, all these other symptoms got worse among people taking the drug; they gained weight and had higher levels of blood pressure, cholesterol, and damage in arteries.

To benefit from bitter melon, it's important to take a good quality extract. Based on my own research and studies around the world, I recommend taking it in combination with the other supplements I've described. The next chapter explains how to put all this information into practice.

CHAPTER 12
The Practical Plan

• • •

THE IDEA OF MAKING CHANGES in one's diet and lifestyle habits can seem overwhelming, but it becomes more practical by looking at simple steps that will put you on a road to better health. The most important point to keep in mind is that there is too much sugar and starch in most foods we eat, as well as too much sugar in many popular beverages.

Sugar in liquids has the greatest negative effect on the glucose-insulin system. Early on in my animal research, I saw that sugar raised blood pressure significantly, but the effect could be reduced if oat fiber was consumed at the same time. No doubt, the fiber slowed down the absorption of sugar, reducing its harmful effect on metabolism. Gelatinous foods, such as the fiber in oats, are especially effective at reducing the sugar effect. I am not suggesting that you continue to drink a lot of sweetened drinks along with oat fiber, or any other fiber for that matter. Rather, I want to emphasize the negative effect of sweetened drinks, which are often consumed outside of meal times.

If you remember the glycemic index from chapter 5, it is best to avoid foods and beverages that rapidly elevate blood glucose — foods that rank high on the glycemic index. While we should try to avoid high-glycemic foods and drinks, if you occasionally want to treat yourself, the glycemic load — the effect of all the components of a meal, combined — can be reduced by having low-glycemic foods, those rich in fiber, fat, and protein, at the same meal.

Where you eat also makes a difference. People are more likely to eat too much when watching television and not paying attention to their appetite. Food is more enjoyable and satisfying when it is eaten sitting down at a table with friends or family.

ALTERNATIVES TO PROBLEMATIC FOODS

Below are a some of the most common foods that significantly contribute to fat gain, insulin resistance, and elevated insulin -- major components of the deadly triangle described in chapter 2. I've also included some simple alternatives.

SWEETENED DRINKS

Sodas, fruit drinks, sweetened coffee and tea, and any other hot or cold drinks with added sugars, which can be many types of sugar, high fructose corn syrup, fruit juice concentrate, or other sweeteners (see the list in chapter 5).

ALTERNATIVES

Water is the best option. If you prefer carbonated drinks, plain club soda or carbonated mineral water provides an option. If you don't like plain water, add a little fresh-squeezed lemon, lime, orange, or grapefruit juice, just enough to add some flavor. An example would be the juice of half a lemon or lime in a glass of water, or about a teaspoon of other citrus juice. Tea and coffee can also be healthy drinks if they don't contain excess amounts of sweeteners, artificial flavoring and/or cream.

STARCHY FOODS

Foods made with refined grains are the ones that most often cause problems, and it's all too easy to eat too many of these. Any type of bread or other baked goods made of refined flour, white rice, and pasta fall into this category.

ALTERNATIVES

Breads and other baked goods made with whole grains are better options. Wild or unrefined rice is another alternative and pasta is available in wholegrain varieties. In addition, it's important to eat these in small quantities, so that they make up a minor, rather than major part of the plate.

SNACKS

The most convenient snacks tend to be the most problematic, as they are often made of refined flour or other sources of starch and often contain sugar. Snacks to avoid include cakes, cookies, pretzels, chips, and candies. Snacking can become a mindless habit, especially when watching television, even when there is no hunger, and then it can contribute to weight gain and health problems.

ALTERNATIVES

A small handful of nuts, fresh vegetables, or a piece of fruit can make healthy snacks, eaten only if you are hungry. These types of snacks can satisfy hunger, whereas those high in starch and sugar are less nutritious, less satisfying, and can provoke the urge to keep eating.

READING FOOD LABELS

Food labels can be confusing if you don't know what to look for, and their format varies in different countries. According to the World Health Organization, the ideal limit for added sugars is 25 grams per day, and the daily total (added and in foods) should not exceed 50 grams for adults and 25 grams for children. Sugar can also be listed in calories, rather than grams. This is how these two measures compare:

  25 grams of table sugar equals 100 calories
  50 grams of table sugar equals 200 calories

When reading labels, look to see how many servings are in the container, and the number of calories or grams per serving. As an example, if one serving of a drink contains 100 calories of sugar, it would provide the ideal limit of sugar for the day. Sugar is also naturally present in some foods, but in the most problematic ones, such as sweetened drinks and packaged baked goods and snacks, this is typically not the case.

  When preparing foods or beverages at home, these measures can be helpful:

  1 teaspoon of table sugar contains 4 grams (16 calories) of sugar
  6 teaspoons of table sugar reach the ideal daily limit
  1 tablespoon of table sugar contains 12.5 grams (50 calories) of sugar
  2 tablespoons of table sugar reach the ideal daily limit

Remember, these are recommended limits for the total added sugar consumed in a whole day, from foods and beverages. To begin reducing sugar intake, take a look at the labels of the foods and drinks you and your family consume most often, and find alternatives for those.

EXERCISE TIPS

Walking is a very good way to start an exercise program and should be a normal part of your usual routine. On five days per week, walking for 30 minutes will produce significant health benefits. Aim to walk at a pace of 100 steps per minute, often described as "brisk walking."

To check your pace, count how many steps you take in 6 seconds and multiply that number by 10. For example, walking 8 steps in 6 seconds adds up to 80 steps in 60 seconds (8 X 10). If that's the top speed at which you can walk, keep doing it and aim to increase the speed. Walking 10 steps in 6 seconds adds up to 100 steps in 1 minute (10 X 10). If you can't schedule a 30-minute walk, aim to walk for at least 10 minutes at a time, a few times per day.

Think about using a pedometer. Wear it on a normal day and see how many steps you take and then, aim to add 3,000 steps to your day. For the longer term, aim to reach 10,000 steps per day.

IMPROVING FITNESS FURTHER

If you already walk or do other types of activity that increase your heart rate, add some resistance training, which improves blood-glucose metabolism. This can be done with weights or by doing exercises that use your own body weight for resistance, such as push-ups and squats.

OTHER PHYSICAL ACTIVITY

The more active you are, the better. In addition to walking or doing other forms of planned exercise, it's helpful to use opportunities to move more during the day, such as taking stairs instead of elevators. Recreational activities with friends or family are another opportunity to be more active. For example, play a game that requires movement when having a picnic, instead of just sitting and eating. Try dancing or playing a sport you enjoy. Or, if you have young children, get up and play games with them.

CAUTION ABOUT SUPPLEMENTS

The expression "dietary supplement' is sometimes linked to the word "scam," consciously or subconsciously. Regrettably, the existence of this association has some merit. A desire for profit leads some companies to overhype their natural dietary products. As an example, there have been advertisements that would make you think that taking chromium would immediately produce a super human in a few days. Alas, even if these scoundrels touted a valid chromium compound, the beneficial effects of chromium take months or even years to be readily discerned. What I want you to remember is that good natural products do exist, but one must use those of good quality, must take an effective dose, and must be compliant with instructions given.

The quality of the supplement is of prime importance and too many times, those of poor quality are easy to find and heavily promoted. In addition to a good quality product, the dose must be correct. Although I believe that most individuals realize that quality and quantity of natural products are important for effectiveness, obtaining the proper information is not always an easy task.

A clinically tested dietary supplement needs to be ingested as directed, every day, consistently. A supplement won't produce the desired results if doses are skipped. Lamentably, humans being human do not always comply with directions. Suffice it to say, even a very effective supplement can appear ineffective if used improperly. I have a saying: "If you don't comply, don't complain."

DIETARY SUPPLEMENT FACTS

Dietary supplements are aids that often improve metabolism and prevent or counteract, to some extent, insulin resistance. Although they are never substitutes for a healthy diet and exercise, they can be extremely helpful in our battle to maintain good health. In the last half century, given the multitude of obesity and diabetes drugs that have eventually produced adverse reactions, it is somewhat surprising that many people are virtually unaware of the potential benefits of safe dietary supplements.

The ingredients described in the last few chapters, and summarized below, are safe ones that I have found to be beneficial and effective in enhancing the proper metabolism of sugars and starches. By doing this, they help maintain healthy levels of blood glucose.

INSULIN SENSITIZERS

Chromium is an essential mineral that helps blood glucose to be used to produce energy, by enhancing the sensitivity of cells to insulin that in turn allow cellular uptake of the sugar without the need to increase insulin levels.

STARCH AND SUGAR BLOCKERS

A white bean extract ingredient, called Phase 2, blocks the absorption of some starch and sugar, and l-arabinose, an ingredient found in plants, blocks the gastrointestinal absorption of some sugar.

FAT BURNERS
An extract of bitter orange, also called Seville orange extract or Citrus *aurantium*, helps to break down fat and slightly increases the number of calories burned by a human body.

BLOOD-SUGAR AIDS
An extract of bitter melon, a tropical fruit, helps to maintain healthy levels of blood glucose.

Each of these nutritional aids work in a somewhat different way and when taken together, the benefits of individual ingredients complement each other. For example, my animal studies have shown that chromium may be more effective when taken with starch blockers, because the blockers reduce the sugar load. The beneficial effects of chromium can be overwhelmed in the presence of too much sugar intake. Some dietary supplement products may contain a combination of these ingredients.

MAKING LASTING CHANGES
The state of our health has been influenced by food and physical activity in the past, and it can be improved in the future with better choices of healthy foods, good exercise regimens, and the proper addition of dietary supplements. However, it's important to recognize, for better or worse, that these effects take time. Anyone who is overweight didn't gain the weight overnight, and losing weight will also take time.

Making some simple changes, such as going for a daily walk and drinking more water instead of soda, can very quickly improve the way an individual feels and if these become habits, they will produce more dramatic changes over time. I encourage you to adopt some of my recommendations: Be consistent in eating healthy foods, be more physically active, and use good supplements as additional aids. This should enable you to move forward on a path to better health.

As I mentioned at the outset, sugar is a "bitter sweet." By understanding its bitter side and how to prevent the damage it can cause, we can enjoy its sweet side as an occasional treat. The sugar crisis is very real, but it can be overcome.

REFERENCES

• • •

CHAPTER 1

World Health Organization. Global Report on Diabetes 2016. http://www.who.int/diabetes/global-report/en/

The State of Food and Agriculture. Food and Agriculture Organization of the United Nations. 2013.

Cohen R. Sugar Love. National Geographic. August 2013.

Tuchman A. Diabetes and the public's health. Lancet. 2009 Oct 3;374(9696):1140-1.

Paton JHP: Relation of excessive carbohydrate ingestion to catarrhs and other diseases. Brit Med J 1:738, 1933.

Aschoff L: Observations concerning the relationship be-tween cholesterol metabolism and vascular disease. Br. Med J 2:1131-1134, 1932.

Himsworth HP: Diet and the incidence of diabetes mellitus. Clin Sci 2:117-148, 1935.

Yudkin J: Patterns and trends in carbohydrate consumption and their relation to disease. Proc Nutr Soc 23:149-162, 1964.

Ahrens RA: Sucrose, hypertension, and heart disease: an historical perspective. Am J Clin Nutr. 27:403-422, 1974.

Yudkin J, Morland J: Sugar and myocardial infarction. Am J Clin Nutr. 20:503-506, 1964.

Yudkin J, Szanto SS: Hyperinsulinism and atherogenesis. Br Med J 1:349, 1971.

Preuss HG: Effects of glucose/insulin perturbations on aging and chronic disorders of aging: the evidence. J Am Coll Nutr 16:397-403, 1997.

Keys A: Coronary heart disease in seven countries. Circulation 41(Suppl) 1970.

Healthy People 2000: National Health Promotion and Disease Prevention Objectives and Full Report, with Commentary. US Department of Health and Human Services Public Health Service, 1991.

Lustig DS. Lowering the Bar on the Low-Fat Diet. JAMA. Published online September 28, 2016.

Kearns CE, Schmidt LA, Glantz SA. Sugar Industry and Coronary Heart Disease Research: A Historical Analysis of Internal Industry Documents. JAMA Intern Med. 2016 Sep 12. doi: 10.1001/jamainternmed.2016.5394. [Epub ahead of print]

Nestle F. Food Politics: How the Food Industry Influences Nutrition, and Health, Revised and Expanded Edition (California Studies in Food and Culture). University of California Press. 2007.

CHAPTER 2
World Health Organization. Global Report on Diabetes 2016. http://www.who.int/diabetes/global-report/en/

Preuss HG, Mrvichin N, Bagchi D, Preuss J, Perricone N, Kaats GR: Importance of fasting blood glucose in screening/tracking overall health. The Original Internist. 23:13-20, 2016.

National Heart, Lung, and Blood Institute. What is Metabolic Syndrome? US Department of Health and Human Services. www.nhlbi.nih.gov/health/health-topics/topics/ms. Accessed September 30, 2016

Preuss HG, Mrvichin N, Bagchi D, Preuss JM, Perricone NV, Kaats GR: Lowering circulating glucose levels that are in the non-diabetic range is important for long-term optimal health. In: Functional and Medical Foods for Chronic Diseases: Bioactive Compounds and Biomarkers. (Ed) D Martirosyan, F Welty, J-R Zhou. Food Science Publisher, Dallas TX 18th International Conference, Boston, MA 18:20-22, 2015.

CHAPTER 3
1. You WP, Henneberg M. Type 1 diabetes prevalence increasing globally and regionally: the role of natural selection and life expectancy at birth. BMJ Open Diabetes Res Care. 2016 Mar 2;4(1):e000161.

Knowler WC, Barrett-Connor E, Fowler SB, et al.: Reduction in the incidence of type 2 diabetes with lifestyle intervention or metformin. New Engl J Med 346:393-403, 2002.

The National Institute of Diabetes and Digestive and Kidney Diseases Health Information Center. Diabetes, Heart Disease, and Stroke. https://www.niddk.nih.gov/health-information/diabetes/preventing-diabetes-problems/heart-disease-stroke. Accessed September 25, 2016.

World Health Organization. Cardiovascular disease. http://www.who.int/cardiovascular_diseases/en/. Accessed September 25, 2016.

World Health Organization. Raised blood pressure. http://www.who.int/gho/ncd/risk_factors/blood_pressure_prevalence_text/en/. Accessed September 25, 2016.

Ahrens RA: Sucrose, hypertension, and heart disease: an historical perspective. Am J Clin Nutr. 27:403-422, 1974.

Preuss HG, Fournier RD: Effects of sucrose ingestion on blood pressure. Life Sci 30:879-886, 1982.

Duffey KJ, Gordon-Larsen P, Steffen LM, et al.: Drinking caloric beverages increases the risk of adverse cardiometabolic outcomes in the Coronary Risk Development in Young Adults (CARDIA) study. Am J Clin Nutr 92:954-959, 2010.

Koren D, Dumin M, Gozal D. Role of sleep quality in the metabolic syndrome. Diabetes Metab Syndr Obes. 2016 Aug 25;9:281-310.

CHAPTER 4

World Health Organization. Obesity and Overweight Fact Sheet. http://www.who.int/mediacentre/factsheets/fs311/en/. Accessed September 25, 2016.

Harvard School of Public Health Obesity Prevention Source Web. Waist Size Matters. https://www.hsph.harvard.edu/obesity-prevention-source/obesity-definition/abdominal-obesity/. Accessed September 25, 2016.

Eriksson K-F, Lindgarde F: Prevention of type 2 (non-insulin-dependent) diabetes mellitus by diet and physical exercise. The 6-year Malmo feasibility study. Diabetologia 34:891-898, 1991.

Tuomilehto J, Lindstrom J, Eriksson JG et al.: Prevention of type 2 diabetes mellitus by changes in lifestyle among subjects with impaired glucose tolerance. N Engl J Med 344:1343-1350, 2001.

http://www.whathealth.com/bmi/chart-metric2.html. Accessed September 25, 2016.

CHAPTER 5

Johnson RK, Appel LJ, Brands M, et al. Dietary sugars intake and cardiovascular health: a scientific statement from the American Heart Association. Circulation 120:1011-1020, 2009.

French SA, Lin BH, Guthrie JF. National trends in soft drink consumption among children and adolescents age 6 to 17 years: prevalence, amounts, and sources, 1977/1978 to 1994/1998. J Amer Diet Assoc 103:1326-1331, 2003.

References

Malik VS, Popkin BM, Bray GA, et al. Sugar-sweetened beverages, obesity, type 2 diabetes mellitus, and cardiovascular disease risk. Circulation 121:1356-1364, 2010.

DiMeglio DP, Mattes RD. Liquid versus solid carbohydrates: effects on food intake and body weight. Int J Obes Relat Metab Disord 24:794-800, 2000.

Akgun S, Ertel NH. The effects of sucrose, fructose, and high-fructose corn syrup meals on plasma glucose and insulin in non-insulin-dependent diabetic subjects. Diabetes Care 88:279-283, 1985.

Hu FB. Resolved: there is sufficient scientific evidence that decreasing sugar-sweetened beverage consumption will reduce the prevalence of obesity and obesity-related diseases. Obes Rev. 2013 Aug;14(8):606-19.

Bray GA, Popkin BM. Dietary sugar and body weight: have we reached a crisis in the epidemic of obesity and diabetes?: health be damned! Pour on the sugar. Diabetes Care. 2014 Apr;37(4):950-6.

Popkin BM, Hawkes C. Sweetening of the global diet, particularly beverages: patterns, trends, and policy responses. Lancet Diabetes Endocrinol. 2016 Feb;4(2):174-86.

Ng SW, Slining MM, Popkin BM. Use of caloric and noncaloric sweeteners in US consumer packaged foods, 2005-2009. J Acad Nutr Diet. 2012 Nov;112(11):1828-34.e1-6.

Sanders LM, Lupton JR: Carbohydrates. In: Present Knowledge in Nutrition (10th Edition), JW Erdman Jr, IA Macdonald, SH Zeisel (eds). Wiley-Blackwell, Ames, Iowa, pp 83-96, 2012.

Jenkins DJA, Srichaikul K, Mirrahimi A, et al.: Glycemic index. In Obesity. Epidemiology, Pathophysiology, and Prevention (2nd ed). Bagchi D, Preuss HG (eds). CRC Press, Boca Raton, FL; pp 212-238, 2012.

Aller EE, Abete I, Astrup A, Martinez JA, van Baak MA. Starches, sugars and obesity. Nutrients. 2011 Mar;3(3):341-69.

American Heart Association. Trans Fat. http://www.heart.org/HEARTORG/HealthyLiving/HealthyEating/Nutrition/Trans-Fats_UCM_301120_Article.jsp#V_nEXuArLIU. Accessed Sept 25, 2016.

CHAPTER 6

Knowler WC, Barrett-Connor E, Fowler SB, et al.: Reduction in the incidence of type 2 diabetes with lifestyle intervention or metformin. New Engl J Med 346:393-403, 2002.

Mitka M. New Dietary Guidelines Place Added Sugars in the Crosshairs. JAMA. 2016;315(14):1440-1441.

Yang, Q. Gain weight by "going diet?" Artificial sweeteners and the neurobiology of sugar cravings: Neuroscience 2010. Yale J Biol Med. 2010 Jun; 83(2): 101–108.

Chia CW, Shardell M, Tanaka T, Liu DD, Gravenstein KS, Simonsick EM, Egan JM, Ferrucci L. Chronic Low-Calorie Sweetener Use and Risk of Abdominal Obesity among Older Adults: A Cohort Study. PLoS One. 2016 Nov 23;11(11):e0167241

USDA. Dietary Guidelines for Americans 2015-2020: Eighth Edition.

Johnson RK, Appel LJ, Brands M, Howard BV, Lefevre M, Lustig RH, Sacks F, Steffen LM, Wylie-Rosett J; American Heart Association Nutrition Committee of the Council on Nutrition, Physical Activity, and Metabolism and the Council on Epidemiology and Prevention. Dietary sugars intake and cardiovascular health: a scientific statement from the American Heart Association. Circulation. 2009 Sep 15;120(11):1011-20.

Vos MB, Kaar JL, Welsh JA, Van Horn LV, Feig DI, Anderson CA, Patel MJ, Cruz Munos J, Krebs NF, Xanthakos SA, Johnson RK; American Heart Association Nutrition Committee of the Council on Lifestyle and Cardiometabolic Health; Council on Clinical Cardiology; Council on Cardiovascular Disease in the Young; Council on Cardiovascular and Stroke Nursing; Council on Epidemiology and Prevention; Council on Functional Genomics and Translational Biology; and Council on Hypertension. Added Sugars and Cardiovascular Disease Risk in Children: A Scientific Statement from the American Heart Association. Circulation. 2016 Aug 22. pii: CIR.0000000000000439. [Epub ahead of print]

Hession M, Rolland C, Kulkarni U, et al.: Systematic review of randomized controlled trials of low-carbohydrate vs. low-fat/low-calorie diets in the management of obesity and its comorbidities. Obes Rev 10:36-50, 2009.

Thomas DE, Elliott EJ, Baur L: Low glycaemic index or low glycaemic load diets for overweight and obesity. Cochrane Database Syst Rev. 2007 Jul 18;(3):CD005105.

CHAPTER 7

Preuss HG, Bagchi D, Kaats G. Role of exercise in weight management and other health benefits: Emphasis on pedometer-based, walking program.

References

Phytopharmaceuticals in Overweight/Obesity Therapy, second addition. (Eds) D Bagchi, HG Preuss CRC.Press. pp 409-416, 2012.

Miller TD, Balady GJ, Fletcher GF. Exercise and its role in the prevention and rehabilitation of cardiovascular disease. Ann Behav Med 19:220-229, 1997.

Ryan AS. Exercise in aging: its important role in mortality, obesity and insulin resistance. Aging health. 2010 Oct;6(5):551-563.

Murtagh EM, Murphy MH, Boone-Heinonen J. Walking – the first steps in cardiovascular disease prevention. Curr Opinion Cardiol 25:490-496, 2010.

Pollock ML, Carroll JF, Graves JE, Leggett SH, Braith RW, Limacher M, et al. Injuries and adherence to walk/jog and resistance training programs in the elderly. Medicine and Science in Sports and Exercise. 23:1194-1200, 1991.

Dishman RK, Ickes W, Morgan WP. Self-motivation and adherence to habitual physical activity. Journal of Applied Social Psychology 10: 115–132, 1980.

Smith AD, Crippa A, Woodcock J, Brage S. Physical activity and incident type 2 diabetes mellitus: a systematic review and dose-response meta-analysis of prospective cohort studies. Diabetologia. 2016 Oct 17.

Tudor-Locke C, Schuna JM Jr, Han H, Aguiar EJ, Green MA, Busa MA, Larrivee S, Johnson WD. Step-based Physical Activity Metrics and Cardiometabolic Risk: NHANES 2005-06. Med Sci Sports Exerc. 2016 Sep 23.

Bravata DM, Smith-Spangler C, Sundaram V, Gienger AL, Lin N, Lewis R, Stave CD, Olkin I, Sirard JR. Using pedometers to increase physical activity and improve health. JAMA 298:2296-2304, 2007.

Richardson CR, Newton TL, Abraham JJ, Sen A, Jimbo M, Swartz AM. A meta-analysis of pedometer-based walking intervention and weight loss. Ann Fam Med 6:69-77, 2008.

Reynolds AN, Mann JI, Williams S, Venn BJ. Advice to walk after meals is more effective for lowering postprandial glycaemia in type 2 diabetes mellitus than advice that does not specify timing: a randomised crossover study. Diabetologia. 2016 Oct 17.

CHAPTER 8

Stein SA, Lamos EM, Davis SN: A review of the efficacy and safety of oral antidiabetic drugs. Expert Opin Drug Safety. 12:153-175, 2013.

Tolman KG: The safety of thiazolidinediones. Expert Opin Drug Saf 10:419-428, 2011.

Wilding J: Thiazolidinediones, insulin resistance, and obesity: finding a balance. Int J Clin Prac 60:1272-1280, 2006.

Mayo Clinic. Glyburide and Metformin (Oral Route). www.mayoclinic.org/drugs-supplements/glyburide-and-metformin-oral-route/precautions/drg-20061991 accessed September 15, 2016.

Low Blood Glucose (Hypoglycemia). National Institute of Diabetes and Digestive and Kidney Diseases, U.S. Department of Health and Human Services. www.niddk.nih.gov/health-information/diabetes/preventing-diabetes-problems/low-blood-glucose-hypoglycemia accessed September 15, 2016.

CHAPTER 9

Schwartz K, Mertz W: A glucose tolerance factor and its differentiation from factor 3. Arch Biochem Biophy 72:515-518, 1957.

Jeejeebhoy KN, Chu RC, Marliss EB, et al.: Chromium deficiency, glucose intolerance, and neuropathy reversed by chromium supplementation in a patient receiving long-term total parenteral nutrition. Am J Clin Nutr 30:531-538, 1977.

Anderson RA, Cheng N, Bryden NA, Polansky MM, Cheng N, Chi J, Feng J. Elevated intakes of supplemental chromium improve glucose and insulin variables in individuals with type 2 diabetes. Diabetes 1997;46:1786-1791.

Martin J, Wang ZQ, Zhang XH, et al.: Chromium picolinate supplementation attenuates body weight gain and increases insulin sensitivity in subjects with type 2 diabetes. Diabetes Care. 29:1826-32, 2006.

Preuss H, Anderson RA: Chromium update: examining recent literature 1997-1998. Clinical Nutrition and Metabolic Care 1:509-512, 1998.

Preuss, HG: Effects of glucose/insulin perturbations on aging and chronic disorders of aging: the evidence. J Am Coll Nutr 1997 Oct;16(5):397-403.

CHAPTER 10

Bagchi, B, Preuss, HG. Obesity: Epidemiology, Pathophysiology, and Prevention. 1st and 2nd editions, CRC Press.

References

Vinson JA, Al Kharrat H, Shuta D: Investigation of an amylase inhibitor on human glucose absorption after starch consumption. The Open Nutraceutical Journal 2:88-91, 2009.

Celleno L, Perricone NV, Preuss HG: Effect of a dietary supplement containing standardized Phaseolus vulgaris extract on the body composition of overweight men and women. Int J Med Sci 4:45-52, 2007.

Wu X, Xu X, Shen J, Preuss HG: Enhanced weight loss from a dietary supplement containing standardized Phaseolus vulgaris extract in overweight men and women. J Applied Research 10:73-79, 2010.

Udani J, Hardy M, Madsen DC: Blocking carbohydrate absorption and weight loss: a clinical trial using Phase 2 brand proprietary fractionated white bean extract. Altern Med Rev 9:63-69, 2004.

Udani J, Singh BB: Blocking carbohydrate absorption and weight loss: a clinical trial using a proprietary fractionated white bean extract. Altern Ther Health Med. 13:32-37, 2007.

Grube B, Chong WF, Chong PW, Riede L: Weight reduction and maintenance with IQP-PV-101: a 12 week randomized controlled study with a 24-week open label period. Obesity 22:645-651, 2014.

Barrett, M, Udani, JK. A proprietary alpha-amylase inhibitor from white bean (Phaseolus vulgaris): A review of clinical studies on weight loss and glycemic control. Nutr J. 2011 Mar 17;10:24.

Preuss HG, Echard B, Talpur N, et al: Inhibition of starch and sucrose gastrointestinal absorption in rats by various dietary supplements alone and combined. Acute studies Int J Med Sci 4:196-202, 2007.

Preuss HG, Echard B, Talpur N, et al.: Inhibition of starch and sucrose gastrointestinal absorption in rats by various dietary supplements alone and combined. Subchronic studies. Int J Med Sci 4:209-215, 2007.

Inoue S, Sanai K, Seri K: Effect of L-arabinose on blood glucose level after ingestion of sucrose-containing food in humans. J Jpn Soc Nutr Food Sci 53:243-247, 2000.

Krog-Mikkelsen I, Hels O, Tetens I, Holst JJ, Andersen JR, Bukhave K. The effects of L-arabinose on intestinal sucrase activity: dose-response studies in vitro and in humans. Am J Clin Nutr. 2011 Aug;94(2):472-8.

CHAPTER 11

St-Onge MP, Gallagher D. Body composition changes with aging: the cause or the result of alterations in metabolic rate and macronutrient oxidation? Nutrition. 2010 Feb;26(2):152-5.

Roberts SB, Dallal GE. Energy requirements and aging. Public Health Nutrition. 2005 Oct;8(7):1028-1036.

Stohs SJ, Preuss HG, Shara M. The safety of Citrus aurantium (bitter orange) and its primary protoalkaloid p-synephrine. Phytother Res. 2011 Oct;25(10):1421-8.

Shara M, Stohs SJ, Mukattash TL. Cardiovascular Safety of Oral p-Synephrine (Bitter Orange) in Healthy Subjects: A Randomized Placebo-Controlled Cross-over Clinical Trial. Phytother Res. 2016 May;30(5):842-7.

Stohs SJ, Preuss HG, Keith SC, Keith PL, Miller H, Kaats GR. Effects of p-synephrine alone and in combination with selected bioflavonoids on resting metabolism, blood pressure, heart rate and self-reported mood changes. Int J Med Sci. 2011 Apr 28;8(4):295-301.

Stohs SJ, Preuss HG, Shara M. A review of the human clinical studies involving Citrus aurantium (bitter orange) extract and its primary protoalkaloid p-synephrine. Int J Med Sci. 2012;9(7):527-38.

Clouatre DL, Rao SN, Preuss HG. Bitter melon extracts in diabetic and normal rats favorably influence blood glucose and blood pressure regulation. J Med Food. 2011 Dec;14(12):1496-504.

Yama OE, Osinubi AA, Noronha CC, Okanlawon AO. Effect of methanolic seed extract of Momordica charantia on body weight and serum cholesterol level of male Sprague-Dawley rats. Nig Q J Hosp Med. 2010 Oct-Dec;20(4):209-13.

Huang HL, Hong YW, Wong YH, Chen YN, Chyuan JH, Huang CJ, Chao PM. Bitter melon (Momordica charantia L.) inhibits adipocyte hypertrophy and down regulates lipogenic gene expression in adipose tissue of diet-induced obese rats. Br J Nutr. 2008 Feb;99(2):230-9.

Efird JT, Choi YM, Davies SW, Mehra S, Anderson EJ, Katunga LA. Potential for improved glycemic control with dietary Momordica charantia in patients with insulin resistance and pre-diabetes. Int J Environ Res Public Health. 2014 Feb 21;11(2):2328-45.

Inayat U Rahman, Khan RU, Khalil Ur Rahman, Bashir M. Lower hypoglycemic but higher antiatherogenic effects of bitter melon than glibenclamide in type 2 diabetic patients. Nutr J. 2015 Jan 26;14:13.

CHAPTER 12

World Health Organization. Guideline: Sugars Intake for Adults and Children. Geneva. 2015.

Tudor-Locke C, Schuna JM Jr, Han H, Aguiar EJ, Green MA, Busa MA, Larrivee S, Johnson WD. Step-based Physical Activity Metrics and Cardiometabolic Risk: NHANES 2005-06. Med Sci Sports Exerc. 2016 Sep 23.

Eikenberg JD, Savla J, Marinik EL, Davy KP, Pownall J, Baugh ME, Flack KD, Boshra S, Winett RA, Davy BM. Prediabetes Phenotype Influences Improvements in Glucose Homeostasis with Resistance Training. PLoS One. 2016 Feb 3;11(2):e0148009.

Preuss HG, Clouatre D. Potential of diet and dietary supplementation to ameliorate the chronic clinical perturbations of the Metabolic Syndrome. In: Nutritional and Integrative Strategies in Cardiovascular Medicine. (eds) S Sinatra and M Houston, CRC Press, pp 148-178, 2015.

AUTHOR BIOGRAPHY

• • •

HARRY G. PREUSS, MD, MACN, CNS, received his BA (3 years) and MD (4 years) from Cornell University, Ithaca, NY, and New York City, NY. He trained for 3 years in internal medicine at Vanderbilt University Medical Center, studied for 2 years as a fellow in renal physiology at Cornell University Medical Center, and spent 2 years in clinical and research training in nephrology at Georgetown University Medical Center. During his training years, Dr. Preuss was a special research fellow of the National Institutes of Health (NIH). Following 5 years as an assistant and associate (tenured) professor of medicine at the University of Pittsburgh Medical Center, where he became an established investigator of the American Heart Association, he returned to Georgetown Medical Center. He subsequently performed a six-month sabbatical in molecular biology at the NIH. Dr. Preuss is now a tenured Professor at Georgetown University Medical Center in four departments: Biochemistry, Physiology, Medicine, and Pathology.

Dr. Preuss's bibliography includes over 250 peer-reviewed, original medical research papers, 220 general medical contributions (chapters, editorials, review articles, etc.), 7 patents, and more than 260 abstracts. Dr. Preuss has written, edited or co-edited 12 books and 3 symposia published in well-established journals. He has two other recently published books: one co-authored for the lay public entitled *The Natural Fat Loss Pharmacy* (Broadway Books/Rodale Press) that has sold over 150,000 copies, and a second co-edited for the academic community entitled *Obesity: Epidemiology, Pathophysiology, and Prevention* (CRC Press), which received outstanding reviews from the New England Journal of Medicine and the Journal of the American Medical Association. A second edition has now been published. The Selected Author Bibliography in the next section lists his published papers relating to the topics covered in this book.

In 1976, Dr. Preuss was elected to membership in the American Society for Clinical Investigations on the first try. He is currently an advisory editor for many journals. His previous government appointments included 4 years on the Advisory Council for the National Institute on Aging, 2 years on the Advisory Council of the director of the NIH (NIA Representative), and 2 years on the Advisory Council for the Office of Alternative Medicine of the NIH. He has been a member of many other peer research review committees for the NIH and American Heart Association and was recently a member of the National Cholesterol Education Program of the National Heart, Lung, and Blood Institute, National Institutes of Health.

Dr. Preuss was elected the ninth Master of the American College of Nutrition (ACN). He is a former chairman of two ACN councils – Cardiovascular/Aging and Dietary Supplements/Functional Foods. After a brief stint on the board of directors of the ACN, Dr. Preuss spent 3 years as secretary-treasurer and 3 consecutive years as vice president, president-elect, and became president in 1998. In 2008 and 2010, he was twice more re-elected president of the ACN, the only person to hold this office more than once. Dr. Preuss is a member of the board of directors for the Alliance for Natural Health (ANH-USA) and was made a member of the ANH-INT scientific and medical collaboration group. Dr. Preuss wrote the nutrition section for the *Encyclopedia Americana* and is past president of the Certification Board for Nutrition Specialists (CBNS) that gives the CNS certification. He was chairman of the Institutional Review Board (IRB) at Georgetown University, which reviews all clinical protocols at Georgetown University Medical Center, for over 20 years. Dr. Preuss is currently chairman of the Scientific Advisory Board for NutraSpace.com. He is the recipient of the Harold Harper Lectureship Award (ACAM), William B. Peck, James Lind, and Bieber Awards for his research and activities in the medical and nutrition fields. His current research, both laboratory and clinical, centers on the use of dietary supplements to favorably influence or even prevent a variety of medical perturbations, especially those related to obesity, insulin resistance, and cardiovascular disorders. Lately, he has also researched the ability of many natural products to overcome various infections, including those resistant to antibiotics. He won, through a vote of his peers, the coveted Charles E. Ragus Award of the ACN for publishing the best research paper in their journal for the year 2006 and the ACN Award for 2010, given to an outstanding senior investigator in nutrition. In 2014, he received three Jonathan Emord Awards for his research in the fields of medicine, nutrition, and integrative medicine and was honored at a special dinner given in his honor by the ACN at their annual meeting in 2014.

SELECTED AUTHOR BIBLIOGRAPHY

• • •

Harry G. Preuss, MD, has contributed more than 700 scientific papers and presentations. Below is a list of peer-reviewed and requested articles by Dr. Preuss that address topics covered in The Bitter Sweet: dietary sugar, glucose-insulin metabolism, and dietary supplements for treatment.

Preuss MB, Preuss HG: Effects of sucrose on the blood pressure of various strains of Wistar rats. Lab Invest 43:101-107, 1980.

Preuss HG, Fournier RD: Effects of sucrose ingestion on blood pressure. Life Sci 30:878-886, 1982.

Fournier RD, Chiueh CC, Kopin IJ, Knapka JJ, DiPette D, Preuss HG: The Interrelationship between excess CHO ingestion, blood pressure and catecholamine excretion in SHR and WKY. Am J Physiol 250:E381-385, 1986.

More NS, Rao NA, Preuss HG: Early sucrose-induced retinal vascular lesions in SHR and WKY rats. Ann Lab Clin Sci 16:419-426, 1986.

Preuss HG, Fournier RD, Chieuh CC, Kopin RJ, Knapka JJ, DiPette D, More NS, Rao NS: Refined carbohydrates affect blood pressure and retinal vasculature in SHR and WKY. J Hypertension 4:S459-S462, 1986.

Preuss HG, Fournier RD, Preuss J, Zein M, Garcia C, Knapka: Effects of different refined carbohydrates on the blood pressure of SH and WKY Rats. J Clin Biochem and Nutrition. 5:9-20, 1988.

Zein M, Areas JL, Knapka J, MacArthy P, Yousufi AK, DiPette D, Holland B, Goel R, Preuss HG: Excess sucrose and glucose ingestion acutely elevate blood pressure in spontaneously hypertensive rats. Am. J. Hyper 3:380-386, 1990.

Zein M, Areas JL, Preuss HG: Chronic effects of excess sucrose ingestion on 3 strains of rats. Am. J. Hyper 3:560-562, 1990.

Zein M, Areas J, Knapka J, Gleim G, DiPette D, Holland B, Preuss HG: Influence of oat bran on sucrose-induced blood pressure elevations in SHR. Life Sci 47:1121-1128, 1990.

Zein M, Areas JL, Knapka J, DiPette D, Holland B, Al-Karadaghi P, Preuss HG: Development of sugar-induced blood pressure elevation after uninephrectomy in a resistant rat strain. J Am Coll Nutr 10: 24-33, 1991

Preuss HG, Zein M, Areas JL, Podlasek SJ, Knapka J, Antonovych TT, Sabnis SG, Zepeda H: Effects of excess sucrose ingestion on the life span of hypertensive rats. Ger Nephrol.and Urol 1:13-20, 1991

Preuss HG, Al-Karadaghi P, Yousufi A, MacArthy P: Effects of canrenone on RRM-sucrose hypertension in WKY. Clin and Exper Hyper A13;917-923, 1991

Preuss HG, Zein M, Knapka J, MacArthy P, Yousufi AK, Gleim GW, Glace B, Zukowska-Grojec Z: Blood pressure responses to sucrose ingestion in four strains of rats. Am J Hyper 5:244-250, 1992

Andrews P, Al Karadaghi P, Memon S, Dadgar A, MacArthy P, Knapka JJ, Preuss HG: Effects of macronutrients on the remaining kidney of unilaterally nephrectomized WKY. Geriatric Nephrology and Urology 2:35-42, 1992.

Preuss HG, Knapka JJ, MacArthy P, Yousufi AL, Sabnis SG, Antonovych TT: High sucrose diets increase blood pressure of both salt-sensitive and salt-resistant rats. Am J Hyper 5: 585-591, 1992.

Preuss HG, Memon S, Dadgar A, Jiang G: Effects of diets high in sugar on renal fluid, electrolyte, and mineral handling in SHR: Relationship to blood pressure. J Am Coll Nutr 13:73-82, 1994.

Preuss HG, Knapka JJ: Sugar-induced hypertension in Fischer 344 and F1-hybrid at different ages. Ger Nephrol and Urol 4:15-21, 1994.

Preuss HG: Interplay between sugar and salt on blood pressure of SHR. Nephron 68:385-387, 1994.

Preuss HG, Gondal JA, Bustos E, Bushehri N, Lieberman S, Bryden NA, Polansky MM, Anderson RA: Effect of chromium and guar on sugar-induced hypertension in rats. Clin Neph 44:170-177, 1995.

Preuss HG, Lieberman S, Gondal J: Associations of macronutrients and energy intake with hypertension. J Am Coll Nutr 15:221-35, 1996.

Gondal JA, MacArthy P, Myers AK, Preuss HG: Effects of dietary sucrose and fibers on blood pressure in spontaneously hypertensive rats. Clin Neph 45:163-168, 1996.

Preuss HG, Jarrell ST, Bushehri N, Oneijiaka V, Mirdamadi-Zonosi N: Nutrients and trace elements as they affect blood pressure in the elderly. Ger Nephrol and Urol 6:169-179, 1997.

Preuss HG, Grojec P, Lieberman S, Anderson RA: Effects of different chromium compounds on sugar-induced hypertension. Clin Nephrol 47:325-330, 1997.

Shi S-J, Preuss HG, Abernathy DR, Li X, Jarrell ST, Andrawis NS: Elevated blood pressure in spontaneously hypertensive rats consuming a high sucrose diet is associated with elevated angiotensin II and is reversed by vanadium. J Hyper 15:857-862, 1997.

Preuss HG: Interaction of genetics and nutrition on hypertension. J Am Coll Nutr. 16:296-305, 1997.

Preuss HG: Effects of glucose/insulin perturbations on aging and chronic disorders of aging: the evidence. J Am Coll Nutr 16:397-403, 1997.

Preuss HG: Effects of diets containing different proportions of macronutrients on longevity of normotensive Wistar rats. Ger Nephrol Urol 7:81-86, 1997.

Preuss HG, Zein M, Knapka J, D DiPette: Effects of heavy sugar eating on three strains of Wistar rats over their lifespan. J Amer Coll Nutr 17:36-47, 1998.

Preuss HG, Anderson RA, Gondal J: Comparative effects of chromium, vanadium, and *Gymnema Sylvestre* on sugar-induced blood pressure elevations in SHR. J Amer Coll Nutr 17:116-123, 1998.

Bushehri N, Jarrell ST, Lieberman S, Birkmayer G, Preuss HG: Oral NADH affects blood pressure, lipid peroxidation, and lipid profile in spontaneously hypertensive rats. Ger Nephrol Urol 8:95-100, 1998.

Mohamadi A, Jarrell ST, Dadgar-Dehkordi A, Bushehri N, Shi S-J, Andrawis NS, Myers A, Clouatre D, Preuss HG: Effects of wild garlic on blood pressure and other parameters of hypertensive rats: Comparison with cultivated garlics. Heart Disease 2:3-9, 2000.

Bagchi D, Bagchi M, Stohs SJ, Das DK, Ray SD, Kuszynski A, Joshi SJ, Preuss HG: Free radicals and grape seed proanthocyanidin extract: importance in human health and disease prevention. Toxicology 148:187-197, 2000.

Tyson DA, Talpur NA, Echard BW, Bagchi D, Preuss HG: Acute effects of grape seed extract on the systolic blood pressure of normotensive and hypertensive rats. Res Comm Pharmacol Toxicol 5:91-106, 2000.

Preuss HG, Montamarry S, Echard B, Scheckenbach R, Bagchi D: Long-term effects of chromium, grape seed extract, and zinc on various metabolic parameters of rats. Molecular and Cellular Biochemistry 223:95-102, 2001.

Ray SD, Bagchi D, Lim PM, Bagchi M, Kothari SC, Preuss HG, Stohs SJ: Acute and long-term safety evaluation of a novel IH636 grape seed proanthocyanidin extract. Res Commun Mol Pathol Pharmacol 109:165-197, 2001.

Preuss HG, Clouatre D, Mohamadi A, Jarrell ST: Wild garlic has a greater effect than acultivated garlic on blood pressure and blood chemistries of spontaneously hypertensive rats. Int Urol and Nephrol 32:525-530, 2001.

Preuss HG, Bagchi D, Bagchi M: Protective effect of a novel niacin-bound chromium complex and a grape seed proanthocyanidin extract on advancing age and various aspects of syndrome X. In: DK Das and F Ursini (eds), Alcohol and Wine in Health and Disease., Annals NY Acad Sci 957:250-259, 2002.

Bagchi D, Bagchi M, Stohs SJ, Ray SD, Sen CK, Preuss HG: Cellular protection with proanthocyanidins derived from grape seeds. In: DK Das and F Ursini (eds), Alcohol and Wine in Health and Disease. Ann N Y Acad Sci 957:260-270, 2002.

Talpur NA, Echard BW, Fan AY, Jaffari O, Bagchi D, Preuss HG: Antihypertensive and antidiabetic effects of whole maitake mushroom powder and its fractions in two rat strains. Molec Pharmacol and Biol 237:129-136, 2002.

Bagchi D, Stohs SJ, Downs BW, Bagchi M, Preuss HG: Cytoxicity and oxidative mechanisms of different forms of chromium. Toxicology 160:5-22, 2002.

Talpur N, Echard B, Dadgar A, Aggarwal S, Zhuang C, Bagchi D, Preuss HG: Effects of maitake mushroom fractions on blood pressure of Zucker Fatty Rats. Res Comm Molec Pathol Pharmacol 112:68-82, 2002.

Talpur N, Echard B, Yasmin D, Bagchi D, Preuss HG: Effects of niacin-bound chromium, maitake mushroom fraction SX and a novel

(-)-hydroxycitric acid extract on the metabolic syndrome in aged diabetic Zucker Fatty Rats. Molec Cell Biochem 252:369-377, 2003.

Talpur N, Echard B, Ingram C, Bagchi D, Preuss HG: Effects of a novel formulation of essential oils on glucose-insulin metabolism in diabetic and hypertensive rats: a pilot study. Diabetes Obesity and Metabolism 7:193-199, 2005.

Preuss HG, Echard B, Polansky MM, Anderson R: Whole cinnamon and aqueous extracts ameliorate sucrose-induced blood pressure elevations in spontaneously hypertensive rats. J Am Coll Nutr 25:144-150, 2006..

Preuss HG, Echard B, Bagchi D, Perricone N, Zhuang C: Enhanced Insulin-hypoglycemic activity in rats consuming a specific glycoprotein extracted from maitake mushroom. Molecular and Cellular Biochemistry 306:105-113, 2007.

Preuss HG, Echard B, Talpur N, Talpur F, Stohs S: Inhibition of starch and sucrose gastrointestinal absorption in rats by various dietary supplements alone and combined. Acute studies Int J Med Sci 4:196-202, 2007.

Preuss HG, Bagchi D, Echard B, Talpur N, Talpur F, Stohs S: Inhibition of starch and sucrose gastrointestinal absorption in rats by various dietary supplements alone and combined. Subchronic studies. Int J Med Sci 4:209-215, 2007.

Perricone NV, Echard B, Preuss HG: Blood pressure lowering effects of niacin-bound chromium in sucrose-fed rats: renin-angiotensin system. J Inorg Bio 102:1541-1548, 2008.

Preuss HG, Echard B, Bagchi D, Stohs S: Comparing metabolic effects of six different chromium compounds J Inorg Biochem 102:1986-1990, 2008.

Preuss HG, Echard B, Yasmin T, Bagchi D, Perricone NV, Yamashita E: Astaxanthin lowers blood pressure and lessens the activity of the renin-angiotensin sysem in Zucker Fatty Rats. Journal of Functional Foods 1:13-22, 2009.

Ifland JR, Sheppard K, Preuss HG, Marcus MT, Rourke KR, Taylor WC, Bureau K, Manso G: Refined food addicition: A classic substance use disorder. Medical Hypotheses 72:518-526, 2009.

Clouatre D, Talpur N, Talpur F, Echard B, Preuss HG: Comparing metabolic and inflammatory parameters among rats consuming different forms of hydroxycitric acid: a pilot study. Current Topics In Nutraceutical Res 6:201-210, 2008.

Preuss HG: Bean amylase inhibitor and other carbohydrate absorption blockers: Effects on diabesity and general health. J Amer Coll Nutr 28:266-276, 2009.

Perricone NV, Bagchi D, Echard B, Preuss HG: Long-term metabolic effects of different doses of niacin-bound chromium on Sprague-Dawley rats. Molecular and Cellular Biochemistry 338:91-103, 2009.

Preuss HG, Echard B, Bagchi D, Clouatre D, Perricone NV: Gel and powdered formulations of Coenzyme Q10 affects various parameters in spontaneously hypertensive rats. Molecular and Cellular Biochemistry 340:169-173, 2010.

Preuss HG, Echard B, Bagchi D, Perricone NV: Maitake mushroom extracts ameliorate progressive hypertension and other chronic metabolic perturbations in aging female rats. Int J Med Sci 7:169-180, 2010.

Preuss HG, Echard B, Clouatre D, Bagchi D, Perricone NV: Niacin-bound chromium (NBC) increases life span in Zucker rats. J Inorg Chem 105:1344-1349, 2011.

Preuss HG, Echard MT, Bagchi D, Perricone NV: Effects of astaxanthin on blood preussure and insulin sensitivity are not directly interdependent. Int J Med Sci 8:126-138, 2011.

Clouatre D, Echard B, Preuss HG: Effects of bitter melon extracts in diabetic and normal rats on blood glucose and blood pressure regulation. J Med Foods 14:1496-1504, 2011.

Preuss HG, Echard B, Fu J, Perricone NV, Bagchi D, Kaylor M, Zhuang C: Fraction SX of maitake mushroom influences blood glucose levels and blood pressure in streptozotocin-induced diabetic rats. J Medicinal Foods 15:901-908, 2012.

Preuss HG, Echard B, Perricone NV: Comparing effects of CHO blockers and chromium on sugar –induced perturbations of insulin sensitivity and BP in rats. J Amer Coll Nutr 32:58-65, 2013.

Preuss HG, Mrvichin N, Bagchi D, Preuss J, Perricone N, Kaats GR: Importance of fasting blood glucose in screening/tracking over-all health. The Original Intern ist 23:13-20, 2016.

Preuss HG, Mrvichin N, Bagchi D, Preuss J, Perricone N, Kaats GR: Fasting circulating glucose levels in the non-diabetic range correlate appropriately with many components of the metabolic syndrome. The Original Internist 23:78-89, 2016.

Preuss HG, Mrvichin N, Bagchi D, Preuss J, Perricone N, Kaats GR: General Lack of Correlations between Individual Age and Signs of the Metabolic Syndrome in Those With Non-Diabetic Fasting Glucose (to be submitted).

Preuss HG, Zein M, Areas JL, Gao CY. Macronutrients in the diet: A possible association with age related hypertension. In Endocrine Function and Aging. Ed. Armbrecht TJ, Coe R, Wongsurawat N. Publishers, Springer-Verlag, New York, NY, pp. 161-174, 1990.

Preuss HG: The insulin system in health and disease (Editorial). JAm Coll Nutr 16:393-394, 1997.

Preuss HG: Aging: relationship to insulin resistance. Maturity: Canada 1:12-14, 1998.

Preuss HG, Bagchi D, Clouatre D: Insulin resistance; a factor in aging. In: Ghen MJ, Corso N, Joiner-Bey H, Klatz R, Dratz A (eds), The Advanced Guide to Longevity Medicine. Ghen, Landrum SC, pp 239-250, 2001.

Preuss HG, Preuss JM: The global diabetes epidemic: focus on the role of dietary sugars and refined carbohydrates in strategizing prevention. In: Metabolic Medicine and Surgery, (editors) MM Rothkopf, MJ Nusbaum, LP Haverstick. CRC Press, Boca Raton Fl, pp 183-206, 2014.

Preuss HG, Clouatre D: Potential of diet and dieatary supplementation to ameeliorate the chronic clinical perturbations of the Metabolic

Syndrome. In: Nutritional and Integrative Strategies in Cardiovascular Medicine. (eds) S Sinatra and M Houston, CRC Press, Boca Raton Florida, pp 148-178, 2015.

Ifland JR, Preuss HG, Marcus MT, Rourke KM, Taylor WC, Wright HT. Processed Food Addiction and Cardiovascular Disease. Revista Factores de Risco. 33:69-93, 2014. (Portuguese)

Preuss HG, Bagchi D, Kaats G, Perricone NV, Scheckenbach R, Clouatre DL: *Garcinia cambogia*: a valuable member of the fat loss pharmacy. The Original Internist 21:207-214, 2014.

Ifland J, Preuss HG, Marcus MT, Rourke KM, Taylor WC, Wright HT: Clearing the confusion around processed food addiction (commentary). J Amer Coll Nutr 34:240-243, 2015.

Kaats GR, Nugent S, Stohs S. Preuss HG: Using a body composition improvement index (BCI) to improve the assessment of nutritional interventions. Current Nutrition and Food Sciences 12...:0-0, 2016

Preuss HG: Bagchi D, Clouatre D, Perricone N: Effects of different dietary fibers on sugar-induced blood pressure elevations in hypertensive rats. Focus on viscosity. In: Nutraceuticals and Functional Foods in Human Health and Disease Prevention. (Eds) D Bagchi, HG Preuss, CRC Press, Boca Raton. Fl. pp 327-342, 2015.

Ifland JR, Preuss, Marcus MT, Rourke KM, Taylor WC, Wright TR, Sheppard K: Functional Foods in the treatment of processed food addiction and the metabolic syndrome.. In: Nutraceuticals and Functional Foods in

Human health and Disease Prevention. (Eds) D Bagchi, HG Preuss, CRC Press, Boca Raton, Fl. pp 43-60, 2015.

Preuss HG, Mrvichin N, Bagchi D, Preuss JM, Perricone NV, Kaats GR. Lowering circulating glucose levels that are in the non-diabetic range is important for long-term optimal health. In: Functional and Medical Foods for Chronic Diseases: Bioactive Compounds and Biomarkers. (ED) D Martirosyan, F Welty, J-R Zhou. Vol 18, Functional Food Center, Dallas TX. pp 20-23, 2015.

www.ingramcontent.com/pod-product-compliance
Lightning Source LLC
Chambersburg PA
CBHW070834310526
45788CB00017B/723